GOODBYE ALLERGIES

Goodbye
Allergies

JUDGE TOM R. BLAINE

The Citadel Press   SECAUCUS, NEW JERSEY

To the medical pioneers,
living and dead,
of hypoglycemia and hypoadrenocorticism,
this book is respectfully dedicated.

PREFACE

When the first edition of *"Goodbye Allergies"* appeared in 1965, many physicians regarded hypoglycemia, or low blood sugar, as a fad and not a disease. Many books on hypoglycemia by medical and lay nutritionists have been published during the past eleven years. The medical journals have repeatedly explained the seriousness of the disease and how to diagnose and treat low blood sugar patients.

Physicians from all over the world have told me how long suffering allergic patients became strong and healthy by following my suggestions. Many of these doctors said they first regarded *Goodbye Allergies* as a worthless writing of a layman.

Thousands of readers from two continents expressed their gratitude for a book they said caused them to recover from years of suffering and misery. The phenomenal sales of the book resulted largely from doctors' and patients' word of mouth recommendations.

I was prompted to write the first edition largely as a result of conversations I had with doctors about the conventional methods of treating allergy cases. I found a general lack of enthusiasm among physicians regarding procedures and results in allergy cases. Most doctors commented on the usual failure of physicians to be able to give more than partial, temporary relief to allergic patients.

The book explains a new, and when fairly tried by physicians and patients, highly successful method of controlling, and sometimes curing, allergic diseases. As might be expected, some physicians still object to any change different from that used 50 years ago in the treatment of these miserable and unhappy people. As Dr. Sam E. Roberts wrote in his newest book, *Exhaustion; Causes and Treatment,* "The *informed* public is now demanding treatment set forth by Judge Blaine. When the public demands certain things, it usually gets them."

Many brilliant and highly skilled physicians have difficulty in expressing medical terms, experiences, and opinions in language easily understandable by laymen. Most of their writings are for medical journals or medical books to be read by other doctors who would be bored by articles written for the general reading public.

What has been done in this book is to take available articles from medical journals dealing with nutrition and the adrenal cortex extract or hypoadrenocorticism plan of treatment for allergic diseases, and rewrite them in language any intelligent layman can understand without having to resort to medical dictionaries and without having to ask for explanations from physicians.

I am deeply indebted to many wonderful doctors who, without charge, gladly helped me obtain medical material relating to hypoadrenocorticism (adrenal cortex insufficiency) and hypoglycemia (low blood sugar), and patiently answered my many questions regarding these subjects.

Even after I wrote the first edition, I could never have published it had not a dozen or more of the nation's greatest physicians read copies of the first draft of the manuscript and given me suggestions and corrections which I incorporated into the text. To these dedicated doctors, not one of whom charged me a reading fee, I shall always be thankful.

Tom R. Blaine

1.

MORE MISERABLE THAN SICK

If you are one of the nearly twenty million known sufferers from allergic diseases in the United States, I bring you a message of hope and cheer. You can be cured of your allergies, or, if not cured, your health can be so much improved that your allergic diseases will cause you little or no concern.

Why am I so emphatic in saying you can be restored to such a marvelous state of health? After suffering from what the doctors called multiple allergies for more than sixty years, I was cured by a diet and medication given me by my family physician. Thousands of other allergy patients in all parts of the nation have been cured in the same manner.

This new treatment of allergies is one of the miracles of modern medicine. It is not a fad; it promotes nothing for sale; it was not thought up by medical charlatans; it does not require the services of a high-priced specialist; the drugs can be administered by your own physician as well as by any other doctor, and the diet can be followed easily.

From my allergists I learned that the word

"allergy" denotes a condition in which the response of an organism alters after contact with a foreign substance. An allergy, then, is an abnormal reaction of living tissues exposed to a specific substance. Yet the offending thing, the allergen, may produce no unfavorable reaction in a majority of people. It is not poisonous or pernicious per se.

The most common type of allergy is hay fever, known medically as allergic rhinitis. Seasonal hay fever is usually caused by hypersensitivity to the pollens of grasses, weeds, and trees at certain seasons of the year. Perennial hay fever may occur at any time or continue throughout the year. It may result from what we breathe, what we eat, drugs, chemicals, and from plants with which we come in contact. We are told we may be sensitive to changes in the weather, sunlight, gas fumes, and many other things. There seems to be no limit to the number of substances that may be harmful to us if we are sensitive to one or more of the known allergens. We may even be sensitive to cold — a physical allergy.

The sting of a bee or a wasp will make me ill. Once, while working in my back yard, I was stung by a wasp and my neighbor, a doctor working in his yard, hurriedly gave me an injection of an antihistamine which soon overcame the allergic reaction.

Fungus spores, the dander of animals (including house pets), feathers, dusts, flavoring and preservative materials, and serums are some of the more common allergens. Practically any food we eat or drink may act as an allergen. Milk, eggs, wheat, and white potatoes head the lists of foods which may cause allergic difficulties.

We have been taught that most, but by no means all, allergens are proteins. We have found from our experiences that we can suffer from asthma, migraine headache, hives, eczema, and many other allergic diseases, because of something we have eaten or inhaled, or because of something with which we have merely come in contact. I was told by a physician that I should avoid silk and woolen materials. I had just been informed by the same doctor that my skin tests revealed I was hypersensitive to so many different foods that I wondered if there were enough foods to which I was not allergic to keep me alive. To make my day perfect, I was told that I might later become hypersensitive to any food I was then permitted to eat!

Usually, allergies are diagnosed by means of a detailed history and skin tests. Intracutaneous injections and scratches are made to determine a negative or a positive reaction to suspected foods, inhalants, and other substances. In my own case, skin tests revealed sensitivity to so many different things that the doctors admitted they were of little value. After years of these tests, I found that the only diagnostic method of any value as to foods was an "off and on" experimentation with many different foods. However, allergy to foods may exist even when skin tests are negative!

After eliminating this and that food from my diet, later adding one and then another of the omitted foods, I found I could not tolerate any food generally known to cause allergies. In addition to those already named, I was not supposed to eat chocolate, several kinds of fruit, peanuts, tomatoes, and certain other foods.

My doctors informed me that if I would drop one of my allergic foods from my diet for a period of months I would become desensitized to it and it would probably cause me no further trouble when I started to eat it again. After years of attempting to desensitize against my enemy foods, the only change I noted, if any, was that I was more sensitive to them than before I had dropped them from my diet.

Doctors have said the histamine released by the sensitized cells, upon our exposure to allergens, causes us to have hay fever, asthma, migraiine, skin eruptions, or whatever manifestation of allergies we may have. Most of us got tremendous temporary relief from our allergic symtoms by taking the antihistamines prescribed for us.

We have found that there is a hereditary predisposition toward allergies; that is, they run in families. We have also observed that when we have some emotional problems, when we are overworked or when things don't go as we expect, our allergies are worse. If we enjoyed a period of time in which there was little stress or strain, our allergic disorders usually improved. The emotional variable has been very confusing to those allergists who believe that contact of some part of our bodies with allergens is the cause of all allergic diseases. Some doctors have theorized that allergies are caused mentally and should be treated by removing the patient's deep-seated emotional problems.

Many of the treatments employed during the past fifty years for people who are ill and sometimes barely able to stay up and around, seem to be rather primitive. For two years I took weekly injections of preparations supposedly made of the particular inhalants and contactants to which I was sensitive. These "shots," I was told, would desensitize me against the pollens, dusts, feathers, and animal dandruffs which caused me so much trouble. After twenty-four months of torture, with no beneficial results, I decided I had enough "desensitization."

About that time, I was given an adrenalin kit and told to give myself a hypodermic injection of adrenalin when breathing became difficult. I returned the kit after having tried to use it for three weeks, stating that I would just as soon be dead as to have to use that needle all of the time.

At another time, my nasal passages were cauterized with some sort of solution which made me feel that a red-hot rod had been thrust into each nostril. My rhinitis, or hay fever, was much worse after the cauterization.

It was suggested to me several times that my allergies probably were the result of unsolved emotional conflicts and that psychiatry might give me some relief. By that time I was so disgusted with the allergists' theories and beliefs that, fortunately for me, I did not waste any of my modest earnings on psychiatric treatment for my allergic diseases.

I know some allergy sufferers who have actually been given shock treatments. Many have undergone useless and unnecessary surgery which only aggravated their allergic conditions and made it more difficult than ever for them to achieve normal health.

You may have the impression this book was written for the purpose of attacking the medical profession. I hasten to assure you that such was not my intention. I was reared with the belief that two people are always right: my minister and my doctor. I sincerely believe that more than 95 per cent of all physicians and surgeons are high-class, conscientious, and dedicated men and women.

Twenty years' experience as a practicing attorney and thirty years as a judge have given me some insight into what goes on in the minds of physicians. I have found they are just as human as the rest of us. This was forcibly brought home to me by a conversation I had many years ago with a physician. We had been talking about why doctors dislike to testify in court cases, and he asked if I knew the reason. I said I knew why lawyers believe doctors hate to be examined and cross-examined in court. "The lawyers are completely wrong," he replied. "No qualified physician has any serious fear of being 'shown up' before a court or a jury. He will be examined on a subject in which he is an expert. The lawyers know next to nothing about what the doctors have spent years learning. In his office or in the hospital the doctor makes the decisions and gives the orders. In a courtroom the doctor is pretty much like any other witness. There are others who make the decisions and give the orders, and doctors don't like to be placed in that kind of role. That is the reason they hate to go to court."

The difficulty with the theories held by many allergists, that we can be desensitized against allergens, or that allergies are produced by mental or emotional disturbances, is this: These theories sound wonderful, but they won't work. Even if such theories had merit, it would be impossible in most cases to identify every food or foreign body to which we are sensitive; and no person, whether he suffers from allergies or not, can lead such a Spartan life that he never is subject to stress and stain, always has his emotions under control, and never allows any incident to disturb him. Even that effort would put him under stress!

A question the allergists have never answered to my satisfaction is this: "Why do only certain people have allergies?" I have read that skin tests show most individuals are sensitive to some foreign matter. Our bodies are invaded by outside substances to which skin tests show we are sensitive, yet, only a low percentage of people develop allergic diseases. It has always seemed to me that if we can find the answer to the above question, we will know the real cause of allergic diseases.

Before I was cured of allergies, I found I could get along fairly well by observing a lot of rules I had learned from a trial and error procedure. Oranges and grapefruit never caused me trouble, but canned citrus fruit juice of any kind gave me plenty of difficulty. On a business trip to southern Texas, I asked a manufacturer of canned juices if he knew why I could only tolerate fresh fruit or hand-squeezed juices. He said it was impossible to manufacture citrus juices without getting some of the ground-up seeds and peel in the processed products. He suggested that I eat some orange seeds and peelings to see what, if anything, would develop. I followed his suggestion and the next day I had a severe rhinitis and an eczema over most of my body.

Milk has always been one of my allergic foods, yet

I always drank it since I felt I had to have its calcium and phosphorus. I was most allergic to pasteurized milk, and a little less sensitive to raw and canned milk. I found a particular brand — dry, powdered, and nonfat — which I seemed to be able to tolerate better than any other kind. Since I had to take antihistamines even with this dry form, I always drank my daily supply of milk at one time. I also drank a prepared soybean milk, since it was supposed to have many of the properties of cow's milk.

I learned that some foods would cause me little or no trouble if taken alone, but would trigger some severe allergic attacks in combinations of two or three. I had to be careful to avoid sudden chills, although I have gotten my voice back many times by breathing the fumes from boiling water containing tincture of benzoin compound, and then taking repeated icy showers.

I think it is generally conceded that there are two basic types of food allergy: (1) fixed type, which is always manifest when the particular food is ingested, and (2) cyclical type, in which the food — if sensitivity to it is mild — can be dropped from use for a long time and then reintroduced into the diet in small quantities and infrequently without giving rise to allergic reaction. (There is only one trouble — it rarely works.)

The target organs of food allergy may be anywhere in the body: skin (eczema); respiratory system (asthma); gastrointestinal (diarrhea, etc); genitourinary (urinary frequency and burning); and others.

Food control of allergies is not new. Coca demonstrated it in the 1920's, as did Rowe about 1931 in his publication, *Food Allergy*. During the past thirty-five years, so many doctors have recognized that allergies may be controlled by diet that this method of treatment now has the aura of tradition.

The plan of treatment later to be presented is a new modification of an accepted medical approach. An understanding of some fundamental medical truths regarding the functioning of the glands is a prerequisite to an explanation of how allergies can be eliminated by diet and medication.

Many allergy sufferers are sensitive to the chemical additives in foods rather than to the foods themselves. Since World War II, sodium propionates have been widely used as preservatives for cheese, bread, and tobacco. The propionates occur naturally in some forms of cheese, such as Swiss cheese. For those who cannot tolerate the propionates, the result is an intestinal allergy in which migraine is common.

If, after having eaten a good dinner in the evening, one should develop an allergic attack after midnight or near morning, he should determine if propionates are causing the attacks. I know a man who frequently, after eating a steak dinner, had a severe migraine about three o'clock the next moring. He recalled that at each dinner preceding the migraine he had used a blue cheese salad dressing. When he discontinued eating cheese, he had no more migraine.

Another friend complained about the onset of hay fever some mornings at five o'clock. She had never before suffered from allergies and remembered that her only change in eating habits was that she had started eating cheese before retiring. When she stopped eating cheese the hay fever disappeared.

As a young man, I often had sores in my mouth, and nothing the doctors prescribed helped to heal them. Several years ago I discovered that the sores were caused by an allergy to aspirin.

Because of my sensitivity to gas fumes, we were never able to live in a home with open gas flames or with an ordinary gas floor furnace.

When I tried to discuss some of these things with physicians, I was usually met with a stock statement that many people have idiosyncrasies, and the best thing I could do was to get my mind off myself and lead as normal a life as possible. When a doctor got around to mentioning my "neurosis" or my "hypochondriac state," I was always ready to look for another doctor.

A diagnostician told me in 1931 that I was suffering from multiple allergies and sent me to an allergy clinic. The early thirties were memorable years for more than the great depression which made earning a living difficult for nearly all of us. It was a time when unadulterated Freudianism was popular with both doctors and laymen. Only about half of the medical schools in America then offered regular courses in psychosomatic medicine; yet doctors who had never taken the equivalent of an advanced course in psychology were diagnosing their allergic patients as suffering from psychoneurosis, and sending them to psychiatrists for treatment.

In 1935, I went to Oklahoma City to see a noted surgeon whom I had known for years, since he came from my home town. I knew he suffered from as many allergies as I did, so my visit to him was primarily to get sympathy. My friend, Dr. Patrick Nagle, said to me:

"You have been to the allergy clinics in Oklahoma and to the big-name clinics out of the state and you are right back where you started.

"Don't make the mistake of running from doctor to doctor, trying to get relief from your allergies. All we can do is to try to help you on a day-to-day basis. You are less of a neurotic than any other allergy patient I have, so forget about neurosis. When a doctor tells a patient he is suffering from a neurosis, you can often be sure the doctor is just trying to cover up his own ignorance.

"Be your own doctor. All we doctors know now about allergies is how to help our patients avoid the causes of their illnesses. I admit it is a crude method of treatment, but until medical science comes up with something better, we will have to continue in this manner.

"My opinion, for whatever it is worth, is that we are treating the symptoms instead of the causes of allergies. You and I will see the day, in all probability, when allergies will be cured. I think it will come through the work of biochemists and endocrinologists.

"I recommend that you make a study of nutrition. We doctors know little or nothing about nutrition; yet it is very important in allergy cases."

Dr. Nagle died of cancer before any cure for allergic diseases had been perfected; his words were prophetic. From the day I talked with him, I was convinced that medical science would eventually cure my allergic diseases.

I always had the impression some time my local doctor would call and say: "Tom, a successful means of curing allergies is now available. When do you want to start your treatments?" The cure was not that prosaic, but came rather dramatically as you will later learn. Not only did I get over my allergic diseases, but I gained dynamic and vigorous health at a time when I was near the Biblical three score and ten years.

It seems to me this would be a good time to take a look at ourselves and see what kind of people we, who are subject to allergies, are. We have been told by our doctors that we have relatively higher intelligence than most people. We are usually rather meticulous in our work — perfectionists who sometimes drive ourselves to exhaustion. Our doctors frequently complain that we do not know the meaning of the word relaxation.

In addition to suffering from our specific allergies, we often are nervous, irritable, and apprehensive, and complain to our doctors of weakness, fatigue, depression, and insomnia, especially after physical, emotional or infectious stress. We are frequently treated for low blood pressure and anemia, usually bruise easily because of capillary fragility, and frequently seem to be either too hot or too cold when others appear to be comfortable. We think we have a fever, only to find that our body temperature is one or two degrees below normal.

Often, the women among us tend to be flat chested, whereas the men frequently have little hair on their chests or on the lateral two-thirds of their legs. We usually have an abundant head of fine hair and, when we arise after a night's rest, a puffiness under our eyes.

There are spells in which are appetites drive us to eat exorbitant amounts of foods, especially carbohydrates; at times we have a terrific craving for sugar or salt. Experience has taught us that our allergies are worse when we eat an excessive amount of carbohydrates, yet we seem to be powerless to resist huge amounts of starches and sugars, or products made from starch or sugar.

Well aware that we should exercise daily, we feel too tired from what we must do to exert ourselves unnecessarily. The typical allergic or hypoadrenocortic patient is lean, although some have weight problems they cannot solve. We are constantly reminded that we should eat less and we know we are overweight; yet we don't get enough energy from the foods we eat — excessive in amount as they may be — to do the things we have to, much less the many other things we would like to do.

Our doctors experiment on us and give us the usual medications for infectious diseases without any resulting benefits. Although we pay doctors better than do the average nonallergic patients, we frequently have the feeling that we are not too welcome in our doctors' offices. What allergy sufferer hasn't at some time heard a receptionist say on the telephone or interoffice communication system: "That Mrs. Brown with her awful headache is here. How do you want me to get rid of her, doctor?"

Most of us believed the miracle drugs of this era would cure our allergies, but in that we were disappointed. We watched, with interest and enthusiasm, the progress medicine was making on all fronts in curing the infectious diseases and felt we were the stepchildren of medicine. Sometimes we have been tempted to believe that we are the forgotten people of medicine.

Some of the wealthier victims of seasonal allergies

are able to go to different regions to escape the suffering of those who cannot afford to change their climate; air conditioning helps many others during the pollen seasons. We benefit by taking vitamin food supplements, but we sometimes find we are sensitive to some of the pharmaceutical preparations out of which vitamins are made.

Dieting has always been boring to me although I have had a weight problem since I was thirty years old. Actually, I never "dieted" until I started the diet which got me over my allergies and gave me real health. Before that, I alternately starved or gorged. The diet I will tell you about is the only one I ever heard of for obese persons that is worth the paper it is written on. If you are inclined to be overweight, this diet will be like something sent from Heaven. You can eat three meals a day, have snacks between meals and at bedtime, and not gain weight. That hungry feeling you have had while trying to lose weight will soon be gone, probably forever.

I am certain you will be as enthusiastic about the diet as I was, and for the first time in your life, you will have the grand and glorious feeling that comes when you realize your allergies are disappearing. You will keep saying to yourself, as I did: "Can this wonderful feeling of well-being be real?" When a friend remarks to you, "I never saw you looking better," you will be glad you are alive and thankful to those pioneers in medical science who made your relief from allergic suffering possible.

2.

YOUR AMAZING GLANDS

Your endocrine system of glands consists of the adrenal glands, the pituitary gland, the thyroid gland, the pancreas gland with its islands of Langerhans, the pineal gland and the sex glands. These glands are also referred to as the endocrine or ductless glands because, unlike exocrine or sweat glands, they send their secretions inside the body.

The pituitary gland is a pea-sized powerhouse attached to the brain stem; one of its important functions is to regulate and secrete our growth hormones. The thyroid gland — resembling a small oyster in shape — is located deep in the throat; it provides chemicals which control metabolism and help us deal with emotional stress. Embedded in the thyroid are the parathyroids, which remind us of BB shots. Most people have four parathyroids, but some have only one and others have as many as eight.

The adrendals, each one above a kidney, look something like mushrooms. Actually, each adrenal consists of two glands, a cove (the medulla) and a casing (the cortex), like a nut and its husk. The adrenals are, in a sense, the "kings of the glands," as we shall soon see.

Little is known about the pineal gland except that it lies in the middle of the brain and has some influence on the functioning of the adrenals. The pancreas is six or eight inches long and resembles a bunch of grapes. Its primary function is to secrete fluids (hormones) which help us digest food. This gland is regulated by and owes its functional tone and vitalitay to the amazing chemical power of the adrenals, which influence many hormones.

Nearly a hundred years ago, a young medical student named Langerhans discovered a group of cells in the pancreas neither connected with nor related to the rest of the gland. Later it was discovered that these cells, or the islands of Langerhans (sometimes called the islets of the pancreas), produce the body's insulin. As described in our next chapter, insulin plays an important part in the successful treatment and cure of allergic diseases.

No one seems to know how many chemicals are secreted by any one endocrine gland. Doctors tell us they have found that the adrenals secrete at least thirty-two chemicals (homones), and the pituitary gland secretes at least a dozen. Each of the other endocrines gives off at least one hormone, probably more.

The pituitary is constantly manufacturing and sending out chemicals to stir up the other endocrines, each of which reacts in the same manner. The command and response signals coordinate, speed up, or slow down our bodily and mental functions; they control digestion, the blood stream, the heart, and all of our thinking, feeling, and perceiving.

One pituitary hormone regulates the growth of an infant into an adult. If there is too little of this hormone, the child is a dwarf; if there is too much, the child becomes a giant. Formerly, when a baby was born with a nonfunctioning thyroid, he was doomed to be an idiot; but now, thanks to the endocrinologists, if a baby is born without a thyroid gland and is supplied regularly with the thyroid hormones of meat animals, he will develop into a normal adult.

The hormones of the adrenal cortex (the casing) are the most marvelous of all. They maintain life; without them we could not live, for they are the prime regulators of the chemical processes which convert what we eat and drink from chemical substances into useful materials for the functioning, repairing and rebuilding of our bodies.

If it were not for these adrenal cortex hormones, the proteins, fats, carbohydrates, and minerals which we ingest could never be converted into energy and body tissues. We know now that the involuntary (automatic) nervous system and the endocrine system work together most intimately.

Suppose the body is under stress. The nerves send a message to the adrenal cores, which then secrete a chemical, adrenalin, into the bloodstream. This chemical steps up heart action and narrows the blood vessels so that the blood can be pushed through them with more force; simultaneously it relaxes and opens the air passageways to the lungs so that more air can reach the lungs quickly. Adrenalin also stimulates the pituitary to send out hormones which cause the adrenal cortex and thyroid to secrete chemicals. Instant-ly this process prepares both body and mind to deal with the stress. It accounts for somewhat superhuman feats of strength and quick thinking and acting in an emergency.

You are already saying to yourself: "All of this is interesting reading and something we should know about our bodies, but what does it have to do with my allergies?" The answer is, it has much to do, not only with your allergies, but with your general health. Soon we will see how weak and damaged adrenals are responsible for your tired, worn-out, irritable, and depressed feelings.

I will explain why your efficiency is so low and your tendency to go to pieces is so great, and how your seeming inability to ever get things done is the result of an unhealthy endocrine system. You will be told how your personality can zoom, how you can regain a feeling of wellbeing and a zest for living and doing things — all by building up the adrenal glands.

Doctors tell us we are as old as our arteries, but I say we are as well as are our endocrines. It is my belief, based on my experience, that the greatest medical discovery of this age, as far as allergy sufferers are concerned, is that weak and diseased adrenal glands (even if inherited) can be made into healthy adrenals by medication and by a diet which does not place too much strain on them. *That, in a nutshell, is the story of this book.* The same things that are causing you to be weak, nervous, depressed, apprehensive, and irritable are causing you to suffer from allergic diseases.

The physicians set out to find ways and means to improve our general health by treating the endocrine system. In so doing (perhaps accidentally — I admit I don't know) they came up with the causes and cures for our allergic diseases.

The credit for the relief of allergic diseases rightfully belongs to those physicians and surgeons who work on the one big remaining frontier of medical science, endocrinology. The endocrinologists, like all great men of science, are very modest. They admit that what is not yet known about endocrinology may be more important than what is known. Still, they have pointed the way to health and strength for millions of us who have despaired of ever living normal and healthy lives.

We must remember that medical science has only lately become aware of the subtle workings and importance of the endocrines. This is not difficult to understand. These glands are in widely separated parts of the body; their appearances are not the same, and their secretions are heavily cloaked by chemical subtleties.

All of the body's other glands have ducts which carry their secretions to the places where they serve purposes; but nature has so well hidden the connections among the endocrines and their cooperative efforts that it is a medical marvel that physicians discovered so much of her secrets.

In the succeeding chapters, I will attempt to show you how these wonderful endocrine glands make and keep us the persons we are, well or ill, and how they determine whether we are pleasant or unpleasant, calm or jittery, energetic or always tired. But most important of all, you will see how simple and easy it is to get and maintain a healthy endocrine system, and how, when this is accomplished, your allergies will disappear!

When, in 1959, my local doctor handed me a medical journal and for the first time in my life I read that *allergies were being cured*, I was so excited I could not leave the chair in the doctor's office until I had read the entire article. It was certainly something different from what I had been told in the thirties and forties, such as: "Your allergies are something you are going to have to live with the rest of your life . . . If you are careful of what you eat and if you avoid pollens and dusts to which you are sensitive, you should live to a reasonable old age . . . There is sometimes a tendency to outgrow some allergies. We hope that will be true in your case . . . I think you spend too much time thinking and talking about your allergies. Maybe more outside activities will help you."

I have no bitterness towards any doctor who treated me for allergies. I got the finest he was able to give and his charges were always reasonable. Without the help of these physicians, I would never have been able to continue in my chosen profession. Certainly, none of them can be criticized for not attempting to find a cure for allergies before the means for effecting the cure were known.

In 1933 one doctor advised me that there was a definite connection between calcium deficiency and my perennial hay fever. He prescribed calcium gluconate wafers, which I took for more than a year until an allergy specialist in Chicago informed me that calcium gluconate was worthless and recommended I discontinue taking it.

Now we are told that low blood sugar is usually accompanied by low serum calcium and that introducing calcium into an antihypoglycemia diet or injecting it into the patient's system hastens recovery from the deficiency. This is always recommended, so I have read, where the tests show low calcium serum.

Also valuable were the warnings the doctors gave me shortly before I went on the diet and took the medication which cured my allergies. I was desperate for any kind of help I could get, since my general health had so deteriorated that I was not certain I would be able to continue my work as district judge in a large district. New oil fields were being discovered in all of the counties I served. Litigation was increasing everywhere in my judicial district. I dragged myself home after a day's work with only one thought, getting enough rest so I could try to do the next day's work. Since cortisone made me feel well, I begged physicians to permit me to take it, but all of them warned me that the hormone could and would do me great harm.

One doctor said the use of cortisone was so dangerous that were I to take any appreciable amount I would have to carry a card stating that I was on cortisone. If I were to be injured in an automobile accident and given medication by someone who did not know I had recently taken cortisone, I might die.

Another physician warned me that if I took much cortisone I might get what he called a "buffalo hump" on the back of my neck and my face could become deformed. I was also told cortisone might cause me to have a coronary thrombosis or, for that matter, thrombosis (blood clot) in any of my blood vessels. There were so many other warnings about serious dangers resulting from the use of cortisone that I completely gave up any thought of taking it.

If the adrenals are functioning normally they need no stimulation to make them secrete cortisone and other hormones. I understand, from what doctors have told me and from what I have read, that the adrenocorticotrophic hormone, ACTH, stimulates the adrenal glands — that it activates tired or nearly exhausted adrenals to produce a little more cortisone. However, the effect of ACTH on weakened adrenal glands — even when administered for a relatively short time — can be very harmful. In large doses, the hormone may produce adverse side effects (hypertension, muscle weakness, moonface, or acne) representing exaggerated physiological response.

Some means other than administering ACTH or cortisone must be employed to permit the adrenals to rehabilitate. They must be given a chance to rest and rebuild.

In the following chapters I shall attempt to explain as best I can how some physicians have discovered and worked out a program of diet and medication that allows nearly exhausted adrenals to regain more tone without ceasing their activities (which would result from large doses of cortisone). I hope this will prove as fascinating to you as it was to me when I was researching all available publications and interviewing as many doctors as would allow me to ask them questions.

Many sins have been committed unintentionally against persons who had one or more endocrine disorders. As we will later see, these people were not informed by their doctors of the cause of their depressed and sometimes despondent feelings.

Since I have been a judge, I have heard more divorce cases than all other civil and criminal cases combined; more than 50 per cent of all cases filed in my courts have been divorce cases. Here is the testimony in a typical divorce case brought before me by a wife: The husband complains of being tired and worn out, is unable to get and keep a job, and has some allergic disorders, but his doctors have been unable to find anything organically wrong with him that should prevent him from being regularly employed. The wife's conclusions are that her husband is lazy, worthless, and a liability instead of an asset. She tells the court that it is enough for her to have to support herself and her two children, and that if she can win a divorce there will be one less mouth to feed.

When the husband institutes the divorce case against his wife, his proof runs something like this: The wife has become a sloppy and indifferent housekeeper who constantly complains of exhaustion. She spends too much time, so her husband says, in bed and doesn't even take good care of her own personal appearance, much less the children. She apparently has lost her interest in living and readily admits that all charges made against her are true — that the doctors found nothing organically wrong with her, that the medicines she took for her headaches and sinus attacks didn't do any good. She realizes she spends too much money for vitamin pills and overeats. She confesses she doesn't know what is the matter with her.

You are ready to say to me: "You are a judge, not a doctor. How can you know what is wrong with these unhappy and seemingly worthless people who go through your divorce courts?" That is a fair question, and I will try to answer it. I insisted on having many of these people take glucose tolerance tests and a complete blood count. When my suggestion was followed and it was found that the husband or wife needed medication and a diet for an endocrine gland condition, it was not long before we had a different husband or wife; a home which had been ready to fall apart at the seams was saved.

In one case the wife was fat, unattractive, and indifferent about her home at the time of divorce. After following a proper diet and taking medication prescribed by a doctor who wasn't blindly prejudiced against a treatment he had never used before, she made a phenomenal recovery in a short time and she and her husband came back to court to have the divorce decree vacated.

As I shall later explain, my studies have convinced me that many of the drinking problems of the husbands, wives, and parents who come to the divorce courts are related to endocrine diseases, either inherited or acquired. Our endocrine glands can make or break us.

Since this is a book dealing largely with the endocrines, I assure you I did not submit the revised manuscript for publication until several reputable physicians had read it and had given me the benefit of their suggestions. The opinions I give about physicians are my own, but any statement in the book regarding diet, disease, diagnosis, medication, or any other phase of medical practice, has the approval of physicians and may be accepted by you as if it had been written by a medical specialist in the subject under discussion.

3.

HYPOGLYCEMIA, A NEW NAME FOR AN OLD DISEASE

Hypoglycemia is a low blood sugar condition, the opposite of hyperglycemia, a condition in which there is excess sugar in the bloodstream.

Hyperinsulinism is a medical term used to describe a condition caused by an excessive secretion of insulin by those parts of the pancreas called the islands of Langerhans. Unfortunately, some members of the medical profession will not accept the term "hyperinsulinism" and prefer to call the condition "relative hypoglycemia." It is interesting to note that in some medical articles the terms "functional hyperinsulinism" and relative hypoglycemia" are use interchangeably. Hyperinsulinism results in a low blood sugar — hypoglycemia. It is the opposite of diabetes — high blood sugar resulting from an insufficient secretion of the hormone insulin.

When the islands of Langerhans cannot produce enough insulin the result is diabetes — too much sugar in the bloodstream. The conversion of foods, especially carbohydrates, into blood sugar or glucose keeps the sugar level high. The principal behind urine tests for diabetes is that when the blood sugar rises high enough, some of it spills into the urine.

Hyperinsulinism (too much insulin — the opposite of diabetes) has been called the hunger disease, the starvation disease, and the fatigue disease. An abnormal hunger, sometimes of a most ravenous kind, particularly for sugar, is often characteristic of a low blood sugar condition. Chronic fatigue is the commonest complaint.

In their book, *Body, Mind and Sugar,* Abrahamson and Pezet said: "Perhaps, hyperinsulinism will in time be known as sugar starvation, for that is what it literally is. Sugar is the fuel of every cell in the body. While most body cells can derive some nourishment from other sources, however, the nourishment of the brain is exclusively glucose."

The last statement explains why we who have low blood sugar, or hyperinsulinism, or hypoglycemia, have so many headaches. Our brains, as well as our bodies, are crying out for nourishment — glucose.

Because diabetes, if not controlled, may result in death, much attention has been paid to high blood sugar by the medical profession. Some doctors estimate there may be three to six times as many sufferers from low blood sugar as there are known diabetics, and yet, low blood sugar continues to be largely ignored by the men and women of medical science. Let me explain what I mean by a striking example: *Gray's Attorney's Textbook of Medicine,* a very fine work consisting of three large volumes, is in every law library and perhaps half of the offices of practicing attorneys in all the states.

In the index of *Gray's Attorney's Textbook of Medicine* we find that the entry for diabetes consists of 85 lines and takes up almost a page. Low blood sugar is disposed of in the text (Sec. 133.15, page 1402) in exactly seventeen words: "Hypoglycemia is a decreased amount of sugar in the blood. These people are usually irascible, undesirable employees."

When I inquired of physicians about the reason low blood sugar sufferers have, for the most part, been tossed into the medical waste baskets, I received no satisfactory answers. Dr. Sidney A. Portis, of the medical faculty of the University of Illinois, believed the difficulty is that the cure for low blood sugar "cannot be packaged, publicized, and sold over the counter in a drug store." Dr. E. M. Abrahamson, a noted diabetes specialist, thought that if low blood sugar could be cured by a miracle drug, or if there were some glamorous manner in which physicians could package and prescribe a cure, the doctors would show more enthusiasm in trying to do something for low blood sugar sufferers. Another doctor I spoke with said, "Frankly, I don't think a lot of doctors know how to diagnose and treat hypoglycemia."

It is difficult for a layman to understand why many doctors seem to have a prejudice against hypoglycemia. If doctors will only think of hypoglycemia as they do other bodily ailments, they will be able to diagnose it more readily and learn how to treat it more effectively.

Although many excellent articles have appeared during the past twenty years in medical journals, explaining why hypoglycemia sufferers cannot eat quickly absorbed carbohydrate foods, *some doctors*

*still prescibe sugar for hypoglycemia, which is the
worst thing they can do since sugar primes the
pancreas to secrete more insulin, thus actually making
the hypoglycemia worse.* Only the well-informed
doctor will treat hypoglycemia with a low carbohydrate, high protein diet. He knows that unless
patients are willing to change their self-indulgent
habits during the time they are being cured, they will
continue to complain of hunger, fatigue, anxiety, and
nervousness, perhaps with crying spells, headaches,
mental confusion, and all kinds of allergic disorders.

It is easier to prescribe antihistamines or some
tranquilizing medicine than it is to go through the
long ordeal of persuading patients to meet the facts
squarely — give up what they have always been taught
were innocent and harmless foods which they prize
highly. With many patients, it will be a long selling
job on the part of the doctor to even get them in a
frame of mind to try to trade some of their supposedly innocent eating and drinking habits for good health.

Let us have a look at the kind of people who are
"usually irascible, undesirable employees." Low
blood sugar sufferers are found in all of the profes-
sions, including medicine. They usually have superior
intelligence and better than average education. They
are the thinkers and the doers of our country. Among
the laboring people, low blood sugar sufferers are the
ones who are highly skilled. You see them in large
numbers among the "white collar" workers, the
writers, the artists, the people in show business, in
fact, in all walks of life. Even when not cured, these
people frequently live to advanced years because they
generally take good care of their health as far as they
know how. Also, as physicians have told me, their

tissues age more slowly than do the tissues of other persons because of their particular body metabolism.

Most low blood sugar patients are ambitious and inherently aggressive, and although they are more introverted than extroverted, they usually like other people. Possibly their strangest characteristic is their refusal to recognize defeat when the odds all seem to be against them. They carry on their chosen occupations and support themselves and their families long after those with normal blood sugar have given up. Their "do or die" determination, once they have made up their minds to do something, is a valuable asset to the physician in helping them to be restored to good health.

We have talked in general terms of the principal complaints of the hypoglycemics. These are by no means all of the symptoms of low blood sugar disease. Doctors have told me these people sometimes feel lightheaded and exhausted. They occasionally lose consciousness if the glucose starvation of the brain is severe. Some of them may have had brain surgery when there was nothing wrong with the brain. Doctors report palpitation of the heart followed by convulsions. While I was suffering from hyperinsulinism I had several insulin shocks. However, I did not know until I had been cured of low blood sugar and had read every article I could find on the subject that the frightening experiences I had were insulin shocks. My doctors thought I might have had some slight strokes. I was afraid they were heart attacks, even though all tests showed otherwise.

There is another blood sugar condition known as dysinsulinism in which the tests may show the patient has alternately low and then high blood sugar. Some members of the medical profession who do not accept the term "hyperinsulinism" and prefer to say "relative hypoglycemia" instead, may challenge the use of the word "dysinsulinism," in describing a condition alternating between low and high blood sugar. I cannot see how it makes much difference what the doctors call these abnormal conditions as long as they are properly diagnosed and correctly treated.

I was introduced to hyperinsulinism in 1950, when I had been assigned to hold court for a week in one of the larger cities of our state. We completed the trial of a jury case on Monday and the next morning I had one of the worst migraine headaches I have ever experienced. The right side of my head had that throbbing sensation (more like a pounding feeling) with which I was so familiar, and I felt sick all over. A local district judge offered to take over my bench since his cases for the day had been settled, and he recommended that I take the day off after seeing his family doctor. I went to my hotel room and tried to sleep, but the migraine pains were too severe for me to stay in bed. I called the judge's doctor and he told me to come out to his office and that he would see me right away.

The doctor's receptionist led me into his office a few minutes after I arrived. I expected him to give me the usual sedative, a prescription for antihistamines, and a short lecture on not being so tense. His examination was brief — a few questions about what I ate on Monday and where the pains were in my head. "I think we can get you over this migraine attack before evening, maybe sooner," he remarked casually. "Your blood sugar level is too low. When we get it back where it should be, you will feel fine. I am going to have my nurse give you three antihistamine tablets and three aspirins. I want you to take two of each of them now and in about an hour or so take the other two. As soon as you can, I want you to drink two or three cups of black coffee with no sugar. Then go to the grocery store, get some unsweetened fruit; dried apricots or dried peaches will do. After you have eaten the fruit, you should take a brisk walk for thirty to forty-five minutes. When you have taken the last aspirin and antihistamine tablet, go to your room and to bed. If you can sleep a couple of hours, you should feel fine."

He asked me if I knew anything about low blood sugar and I confessed that I knew nothing about it. He said that his wife had migraine and he had found the plan recommended to me beneficial to her. "What has happened," he said, "is that you have eaten too much carbohydrate, especially sugar. A part of your pancreatic gland is too sensitive; when you eat starch or sugar or both, too much insulin is produced in response to your body's demand and it literally eats up your blood sugar, or glucose. This is why migraine sufferers are nearly always hungry. Your blood sugar is deficient and you feel terrible. It is the suddenness of the fall of the blood sugar which brings on migraine. Everything I have told you to do should raise the level of your blood sugar. The fruit you eat will be absorbed slowly, not fast enough to bring about a lot more insulin secretion."

"Doctor," I asked, "you mean this terrible head-ache wasn't caused by some stress or strain, as I have been told by doctors all these years?" "Oh, stress and strain do have some effect on the pancreas and cause more insulin to be secreted," he answered. "But I don't think migraine can always be classed as an emotional ailment. I can see how easy it would be for one suffering from migraine to become emotional."

I mentioned to him that I usually had a premonition that I was going to have a migraine attack. "This premonition you talk about is caused by the chemical changes taking place in your body. You remember how you felt before you had an attack in the past. Somewhere along the line, before your brain gives that distress signal that it isn't getting enough glucose you know from past experiences you are going to have a migraine. My patients don't all experience for the same length of time the warnings that all is not well with the blood sugar."

After drinking the coffee, taking the medicine, eating the fuit, and finishing the walk, I went to my hotel room. In a few minutes I was sleeping and did not wake up for nearly three hours. When I got up, I felt wonderful but hungry. I celebrated my first real victory over migraine by going out and eating the biggest steak I could find. After that, when I knew a migraine was coming, I followed the same routine the doctor had recommended and always got over the headaches before they wore me out. Before I learned about low blood sugar, a migraine headache sometimes lasted two or three days.

Since coffee is not on the hypoglycemic's diet, you may wonder why it was prescribed for migraine, which is a severe hypoglycemic attack. The pain of a migraine is so severe, and the suffering so great, that ordinary pain killers are wholly ineffective; the sufferer cannot wait several hours for blood sugar to gradually find its way into his bloodstream. Caffeine causes elevation of the blood sugar level soon after it is taken, and also stimulates the adrenal glands to release adrenalin, which helps smother the excessive insulin in the blood-stream.

Under normal circumstances, a hypoglycemic does not drink coffee because he does not want the supply of glycogen stored in his liver (and available as glucose or blood sugar in an emergency) dissipated by caffeine. Neither does he desire to stimulate his adrenal glands to produce more adrenalin.

Any person who has ever experinced a severe migraine will agree that it is not a normal circumstance and that emergency measures for relief are always justified. The migraine sufferer needs blood sugar and adrenalin released into his bloodstream as quickly as it can be done.

One patient told me that when he felt an attack coming on, he drank several cups of strong black coffee and ate two or three pieces of hard sugar candy. I inquired if the candy caused him any bad aftereffects. "Yes," he said, "I am certain it causes me to feel more knocked out the next day, but it helps me get over the migraine quicker." I tried taking candy once with a severe migraine and I thought the sugar made the pain worse and the attack harder to overcome.

What we have been discussing is hypoglycemia which readily responds to a high protein, medium fat, low carbohydrate diet, and the medication recommended in the next chapter. The tests for hypoglycemia are the same as those for hypoadrenocorticism. If it is determined that a patient is not suffering from hypoglycemia but has hyperinsulinism resulting from a tumor or a growth on the islands of Langerhans, surgery is the only effective way to a cure.

I will say without equivocation that there have been more mistakes made in diagnosing the ailments of the people I have known who had low blood sugar than in diagnosing the ailments of any other similar number of ill persons. They have been operated on and treated for about every disease on record. Since all such treatments are ineffective for a low blood sugar condition, there has always remained the "hysteria" or the "neurosis" diagnosis to fall back on.

These wretched, unfortunate, badly treated, but worthwhile men and women deserve more consideration from our well-intentioned doctors than they have been getting. These people, with their higher intelligence, their superior abilities, their determination to succeed when others would have given up, their high ideals, their loyalties to their families, and their willingness to conform to the requirements of our society, cannot be cast aside medically as if they were an unimportant segment of our population. They constitute the backbone of this country. It is imperative that they be cured as it is that diabetics be permitted to live long, useful, and healthy lives.

The diet for low blood sugar must be one that will depress the already oversensitive islands of Langerhans. As we shall later see, it must be one that places as little strain as possible on the endocrines, particularly the adrenals. It must be high in protein but low in carbohydrates, and it must contain only those carbohydrates that are slowly absorbed. Remember, we are trying not to arouse the insulin-making islets of the pancreas. We must "slip up on" these islets of the pancreas with our carbohydrates.

Fats do not increase the activity of the insulin-making parts of our bodies, but we must be reasonable in our intake since excessive fats cause obesity, arteriosclerosis, and diabetes, so our doctors tell us. We certainly do not want to bring on any more ailments than we already have. Since we are trying to cure cell starvation, even when we are overweight, it is better that we eat frequently rather than depend on the conventional three meals daily.

On arising in the morning after a long fast, someone with low blood sugar will not have much pep or enthusiasm for the day's work. Coffee stimulates the adrenal cortex to produce more hormones and these hormones cause the liver to convert its glycogen into glucose; so, we get a lift from an early cup of coffee. The lift is of short duration, for the islets of the pancreas produce more than enough insulin to eat up, as it were, the glucose set free by the caffeine in the coffee; we need another cup of coffee while the liver's supply of stored glycogen is being dissipated by the insulin. Sugar gives us the same stimulating effect; but the glucose coming from the sugar meets the same fate as does the glucose coming from the liver's stored glycogen. What is even worse, the blood sugar (glucose) which was in the bloodstream before we ate the sugar or drank the coffee is used by the insulin, and our blood sugar drops lower than it was before we drank the coffee or ate the sugar.

As you have already found from your experiences, and as appears logical from what has been said, one with hyperinsulinism usually feels best after eating a good dinner in the evening.

Here is the diet I was on while being cured of my allergic diseases:

ANTIHYPOGLYCEMIA DIET

Foods Allowed:

All meats, fish, and shell fish.

Dairy products — eggs, milk, butter and cheese.

Also recommended — 1 pint to 1 quart of acidophilus milk daily.

Milk between meals; milk, cheese and/or butter and saltines before retiring.

All vegetables and fruits not listed below.

Salted nuts (excellent between meals).

Sugar-free peanut butter.

Protein bread.

Soybeans and soybean products.

Decaffeinated coffee, weak tea, and sugar-free sodas.

Saccharin or other substitute for sugar.

Foods to Avoid:

Potatoes, corn, macaroni, spaghetti, rice.

Pie, cake, pastries, sugar, candies.

Dates and raisins.

Cola and other sweet soft drinks.

Alcohol in all forms.

Coffee and strong tea.

All hot and cold cereals (except occasionally oat meal).

Having milk or fruits between meals is advisable in order to prevent blood sugar levels from slackening off (as is prone to occur two or three hours after meals). Ordinarily there is no restriction on salt intake; in fact, many doctors advise low blood sugar patients to take supplementary salt tablets, especially during hot weather, to replace the loss caused by perspiration.

The importance of adhering to this diet strictly cannot be overemphasized. Dietary indiscretions will cause a return of the hateful symptoms of a low blood sugar condition and the accompanying allergic disorders. Unless one has made up his mind to be cured of hypoglycemia and to stick with this diet at all times until the allergies are gone for good, he will be wasting the time of his doctor and his own time in starting the diet.

Probably the greatest difficulty is giving up coffee, but this is imperative. No intoxicating beverage of any kind in any amount may be taken. We must never forget that one of the reasons for following the diet and abstaining from alcohol or other intoxicants is to maintain the blood sugar at a proper level. What we must achieve is an appropriate balance between the sugar-repressing actions of the islands of Langerhans and the sugar-releasing functions of the hormones from the adrenal cortex. We should also remember that some of the hormones secreted by the adrenals actually smother the excessive insulin of the islets of the pancreas when we suffer from hyperinsulinism.

I appreciate the fact that diagnosis of hypoglycemia is not a cut and dried process with physicians. I also understand that many doctors, otherwise well qualified, have not had extensive training in endocrinologic precepts. The symptoms and complaints of the patients are generally vague and indefinite. A patient will tell his physician he is suffering from sinus trouble, severe headaches, or abdominal pains. The doctor knows the patient came to him for treatment for his sinus difficulty, his headaches or his abdominal pains, and too frequently the doctor tries to treat the particular part of the body about which complaint is made. As a layman who has experienced most of the problems of health discussed in this book and was finally restored to robust health, I think the greatest weakness of modern day physicians is their tendency to consider any illness which is difficult to diagnose as emotional and then attempt to treat the patient accordingly.

I tried to get relief from my migraine headaches from at least ten doctors, and all of them 'talked about my reaction to stress. They were right in one sense; my reaction to stress was poor because of inadequate hormone production by my adrenals and an excessive hormone production (of insulin) by the islets of my pancreas. I accidentally went to a physician who knew why my reaction to stress was not good because of special studies he had made to assist his wife in getting over migraine attacks.

Physicians, however, had this advantage: even a perfunctory questioning of hypoglycemics will disclose they all have a myriad of common complaints, such as fatigue, weakness, depression, insomnia, nervousness, and apprehensiveness. They will all say these symptoms are much worse following physical, emotional, or infectious stress.

4.

HYPOADRENOCORTICISM — YOU MAY HAVE IT

The late Dr. John W. Tintera, an outstanding endocrinologist, defined hypoadrenocorticism as encountered in allergy cases as "subclinical Addison's disease." Addison's disease is a disease of the adrenal cortex characterized by extremely low blood sugar. It is not common, fortunately, but until comparatively recent years was considered incurable. Persons suffering from this disease acquire a dark pigmentation of the skin, suffer from low blood pressure, have weak muscles, and frequently are emaciated. The word "subclinical" usually denotes a period prior to the appearance of manifest symptoms in the evolution of a disease.

Recently I read a very old medical book on endocrinology, and it stated that one hormone, adrenalin, was secreted by the adrenal cortex. I mention this to show how much progress has been made in medicine the past 60 or 70 years in understanding the role the adrenal cortex plays in the health, or lack of health, of all of us.

Patients suffering from hypoadrenocorticism have feelings of weakness, fatigue, and faintness practically identical with those discussed in the preceding chapter. Dr. Sidney A. Portis reported, after examining many business executives, that hypoglycemia is definitely related to emotional stress. (See *Journal of the American Medical Assoc.*, Dec. 2, 1950). The consensus of those physicians who have made extensive studies of hypoadrenocorticism and emotional instability, is that the emotional instability is functional in nature and directly attributable to the hypofunction of malfunction of the adrenal cortex.

Dr. Tintera worked out a splendid threefold program for attacking hypoadrenocorticism. He beilieved that patients are always subject to various stresses, and that they should be told by their doctors how harmful dietary indiscretions, fatigue, worry, and intoxicating liquors are. According to Dr. Tintera, the patients must receive from their physicians complete but simple explanations of the nature of their illnesses; the patients will try to adjust their activities and keep on the prescribed diet more willingly if they understand how emotional upsets can produce the hated symptoms and how excessive eating of carbohydrates can put an end to a period of well-being and bring about a return of weakness and fatigue.

This, briefly stated, was Dr. Tintera's program, as he explained it in several articles appearing in the medical journals:

1. *Adjustment of the patient's activity*

These patients must be taught to take environmental and emotional stress in stride. Frequently, their ideas and attitudes must be changed. This is no easy thing to do, particularly with older people. As Dr. Tintera stated, "This aspect of treatment is most important and probably most difficult to achieve quickly and successfully." Merely to tell patients to take stress in stride and then expect a dramatic result would be either idle or naive.

If we want to change their ideas and attitudes, we must go to a deeper level; we have to inquire about the "why" of their ideas and attitudes. We cannot always believe what they tell us, but we have made the first attempt. Maybe we can get at the motivation — one answer to the "why." Then we may have a look at the familial and economic setting. There will be perhaps a dozen other ways to try to find what we set out to learn about these people.

If we can get them to change their ideas and attitudes, increase the widths of their horizons, experience the adventure of getting out of some of their timeworn grooves — in short, get them to live and to want to live — they will not, at least, be early candidates for senility. As it is, most people are shallow at best.

Many of these people have already worked out routines which help them control their emotions. They will learn quickly that they can avoid hypoglycemic reactions by eating less at meal times and by taking snacks between meals and at bed time. They must all be taught that eating candy or any food with sugar is completely out.

I anticipate that someone who has been reading health fad ads is going to ask: "How about taking raw sugar? Will that do any harm?" The best answer to that question was a statement by Dr. Cora Miller of the Greater Los Angeles Nutrition Council: "The only thing of importance that white sugar lacks and raw sugar contains is dirt."

2. *Drug therapy*

The primary aim of drug therapy is to put the adrenal cortex at rest temporarily to allow the cells to return to a functioning state so they will subsequently be able to respond normally to stress. Therapy consists of injections of adrenal cortex extract.

These injections, manufactured from the adrenals of young domestic animals, are given frequently at first. As adrenal cortex sufficiency improves, the frequency of the injections is diminished. Ultimately, provided he has cooperated by dieting properly and avoiding undue emotional exertion, the patient will progress satisfactorily without any further injections. Sometimes, however, a periodic checkup may indicate that the injections of the adrenal cortex extract should be temporarily resumed.

Please do not get the idea that you will have to receive these injections the rest of your life. Whenever your weakened and impaired adrenal glands are put into proper working condition, the drug therapy can be discontinued. No doctor can tell you how long that will take. It may only be a few months or it may be a year or more. As you have already determined from what you have read, the seriousness of the impairment of your adrenals, the control you maintain over your emotions, and the steadfastness with which you stick to the diet, will determine the length of time you will have to take these "shots."

The use of the whole adrenal cortex extract (usually made from the adrenals of young beef cattle) in the treatment of adrenal disease has been neglected by the medical profession since the development of cortisone and ACTH. I am sure the reason is that cortisone and ACTH act much faster than does the adrenal cortex extract.

The new method of treating allergic conditions as related to an adrenal cortical insufficiency recognizes that the patient is an ill person who needs to be treated as such rather than symptomatically. The óverall result is not only relief from allergies, but also an improvement in the patient's general health. Treatment with the whole adrenal cortex extract aims at restoring normal bodily functions. Individual steroids, such as cortisone, hydrocortisone and the like, give dramatic temporary relief but may profoundly suppress the function of the adrenals in addition to producing side effects. Such drastic action is not necessary when dietary regimen supports the effect of the adrenal cortex extract.

3. Diet

The diet for the hypoadrenocortical state is the same as that recommended for hypoglycemia and given you in the previous chapter.

We must not forget that what is attempted in the cure of hypoadrenocorticism is the restoration of weak, semiexhausted adrenals to normal health. The high protein, medium fat, low carbohydrate diet has been found to place the least amount of strain on the adrenals. The adrenal cortex extract injections give the glands a rest and allow them to recuperate while the hormone supplements look after the body chemistry. Physicians have known for some time that our adrenal glands will "beat back" from weakness and sometimes from disease if given an opportunity to do so.

The purpose of Dr. Tintera's three-point program was, in summary, to recondition the endocrine glands — particularly the adrenals and the pancreas, with its islands of Langerhans — to secrete their hormones in sufficient amounts and proper proportions.

Dr. Tintera noted that most allergics have poorly functioning adrenals and that their allergic diseases generally respond to a treatment which puts the adrenals into proper working order. He explained why some of us — sensitive to this, that, and the other substance — suffer so much from allergies, while others are not affected sufficiently by any foreign substance to cause any allergic woes: "Endocrinology has now gotten deep below the end results of allergic processes. In learning about the intricate and subtle chemistry of the adrenal glands, it discovered that the difference between the non-allergic majority and the allergic minority was the difference between strong, alertly responsive adrenals which can and do marshal the body's defenses in a flash, and weak, sluggish glands which are incapable of doing what they should."

In order to understand why one man's food is another man's poison, or stated another way, why over 170 million Americans are not made ill by the invaders which make nearly 20 million Americans miserable, and often at least temporarily disabled, we must remember two things:

(1) The central command post of our body's defenses is our adrenals, and,

(2) Body chemistry is exceedingly intolerant of all substances but its own. Foreign substances gen-

erally are broken down and converted chemically — animal proteins into human proteins, vegetable carbohydrates into human carbohydrates, and so forth.

Some foreign substances like bacteria have to be killed, or at least prevented from multiplying; otherwise we would die of infections. Other foreign substances have to be neutralized chemically and made harmless. These are the substances which cause allergies if the body chemistry cannot neutralize them.

In most persons, the bodily defenses are adequate in warding off any attack by outside substances, such persons do not suffer from allergies. Without the assistance of the hormones from the adrenal cortices, however, there can be no adequate defense. If the adrenals are underfunctioning, or if they are partially exhausted, they cannot fully respond to stimulation and the essential adrenal cortex hormones they produce are insufficient in amount and chemically out of balance with the rest of the endocrine system.

When grass or weed pollen to which you are sensitive enters through the nostrils or mouth, you have hay fever; when your defense mechanism fails in the lining of your stomach, you have some kind of food allergy, perhaps hives; if it occurs in the skin, you have a rash or eczema.

On the other hand, if your adrenals are up to par, you will probably never realize that any of these foreign substances invaded your body. If you were born with weak adrenals, in all probability you have suffered from one or more allergic diseases all of your life.

A person with very poor adrenals may live such a

sheltered life, free from stress or strain, that he will never have allergic disorders. But who would want to live such a life, even if possible? Without stress or strain we would have little or no pleasure in living.

The hormones from the adrenal cortex prepare the body to withstand stress, and if the adrenals are not strong and healthy at birth, and if they are not strengthened by diet, drugs (such as adrenal cortex extract), and the avoidance of unnecessary stress, the whole body will some day be in trouble.

Fortunately, most Americans are born with adrenals of apparently super strength. The reason I say this is that the American diet is bad enough to tear down adrenals with any degree of weakness. The amazing thing is how the most perfect adrenal glands withstand the onslaught of the common American diet.

Many of us drink ten or fifteen cups of coffee daily. Our meals are loaded with sugar and starches. We drink sugared cola drinks loaded with caffeine between meals. If we attend an evening meeting of any kind, there are the inevitable coffee and sweets of some type.

Did you ever observe what the ladies serve when they get together for a meeting? Most of them will be talking about how hard they have been dieting to take off some pounds, yet the food served will be rich in calories from sugar, starch, and fat, and everyone will be expected to drink more than one cup of coffee.

Go to your school cafeteria and see what your youngsters are eating and drinking. Sugars and other quickly absorbed carbohydrates often constitute the main part of their noonday meals. The handy dispensing machines for purchasing sweetened drinks, including cola, frequently furnish our children with more liquid than do the cold water fountains.

I was pleased to read the following statement from the *American Medical Association's Council on Food and Nutrition*, issued June 30, 1962:

> Every effort should be expended to encourage students to adopt and enjoy good food habits.
>
> The availability of confections and carbonated beverages on school premises may tempt children to spend lunch money for them and lead to poor food habits. Their high energy value and continual availability are likely to affect children's appetites for regular meals.
>
> Expenditures for carbonated beverages and most confections yield a nutritional return greatly inferior to that of milk, fruit and other foods included in the basic food groups.
>
> In view of these considerations, the council is particularly opposed to sale and distribution of confections and carbonated beverages in school lunch rooms.

Endocrinologists have told us that the hormones from our adrenal cortices and the hormones from the medulla are so important that without them life is impossible. The adrenal hormones regulate the chemical conversion of food into fuel and building materials. They regulate the transportation of fuel throughout the body for "burning" with oxygen in each and every tissue, and the transport of the building materials. They regulate the transportation of fuel throughout the body for "burning" with oxygen in each and every tissue, and the transport of the building materials and its uses in repairing and replacing cells and tissues.

The greatest break for allergy sufferers, with their weak and poorly functioning adrenals, *is the established medical fact that the adrenal glands have recuperative power*. Without this, the millions who have known the agonies, and sometimes the despair, of allergic diseases would have little hope of a better tomorrow.

Should one ever attempt to cure his allergies by dieting and taking the adrenal cortex extract injections without first seeing a physician for an examination and tests? The answer is a definite and emphatic No. However, you will find the examination and tests are not as complicated and expensive as you may have anticipated. Most doctors who treat allergic patients by diet and the glandular therapy require a thorough endocrine history and a physical examination before making tests, which consist of a glucose tolerance test, a complete blood count, a protein bound iodine test, and a urine analysis.

Some physicians, so I am told, insist on a more elaborate series of laboratory tests to determine the status of the adrenal function. Generally, however, doctors say the minimal testing shown above is thoroughly adequate for detecting any dysfunction.

Not all doctors use the same glucose tolerance test. A six-hour glucose tolerance test is perhaps more widely used than any other.

As far as I know, no doctor permits his patients to drink coffee while following the diet and getting the adrenal cortex extracts. Physicians, however, are not agreed on the necessity of excluding tobacco during such time. I believe I can safely say all of them agree that no patient should smoke early in the morning before breakfast and that smoking should be kept in moderate bounds. Some doctors forbid smoking altogether, others discourage smoking, particularly excessive smoking, and others permit a moderate amount of smoking.

It is my opinion that when our doctors and the general public awake to the necessity for every allergic victim to be tested for hypoadrenocorticism, there will come, out of the research centers somewhere in America, the discovery of a cheap drug that can be taken by mouth and have the same efficiency as the adrenal cortex extract injections.

5.

YOU CAN'T
ARGUE AGAINST SUCCESS

Before I heard that allergies were being cured by diet and adrenal cortex extract, six wholly unrelated incidents convinced me that my adrenal glands were in some way involved in all of the many allergic diseases from which I have suffered. These are, in the order of their happening:

1. In 1921, I was present when a business establishment was robbed by a masked bandit and later the same year I happened to be on a public street in close proximity to a gunfight between police officers and some men who had just committed a robbery. Three men were killed in the battle of bullets. To say that I was frightened on both occasions is a gross understatement. After each incident, I observed my usually stopped-up nose was open and my breathing was free and easy. A doctor's explanation of why the breathing was so much easier through my nose and mouth was that the fright caused my adrenal glands to be overactive for the time being. What happened beyond that he said he had no way of knowing; evidently it was

due to some kind of body chemistry which he admitted he did not understand.

2. I have already mentioned the adrenalin kit I was given by an allergist in the early thirties and told to use when I had breathing difficulties.

3. In 1939, there was a lot of publicity about a vitamin, pantothenic acid, which was supposed to stop hair from becoming gray. Like many other vain people, I purchased a bottle of these tablets, hoping they would prevent my hair from changing its color. I discovered that the vitamin tablets caused me to feel considerably better than I felt before taking them.

I wrote a letter to the manufacturer of the product, a reliable pharmaceutical house, and asked for an explanation for the favorable effect. I received a long letter from the company, stating, among other things, that pantothenic acid is involved in adrenal function. The letter quoted some doctor as having referred to the close correlation of this particular vitamin with the adrenal cortex.

4. In 1940, I went on a candy bar spree one evening, eating at least a dozen candy bars loaded with sugar. The next morning I had a hangover, exactly as if I had been grossly intoxicated the night before, even though I had taken no liquor of any kind. I had a terrible headache; I was weak, shaky, and nervous. I went to a doctor and told him what I had done and how I felt. He remarked: "If you had taken enough liquor to put you in that shape, I would have given you a shot of adrenal cortex extract. All I can do, however, is to tell you to go home and to bed and lay off the sugar." I asked the doctor if this drug he talked about was harmful. He assured me it was perfectly

harmless, but said its effect on allergics was not known. When I begged him to give me some of the adrenal cortex extract, he told me again that he didn't think it would do me any good and that it was expensive. I insisted on taking the maximum dosage, 10 cc., intravenously. In order to get rid of me, I suppose, he gave me the injection — all the contents of a small glass vial. Within a few hours I was over my hangover and felt fine. When I reported this to the doctor, he said he was astonished that the extract had worked so well and so quickly. I am not certain he believed me when I told him it was an overload of candy that had knocked me out.

5. In 1957, I took a vacation trip in the New England states. Before starting east, I packed a large bottle of antihistamine tablets, since I knew I would be eating shell seafoods nearly every day. This medication may have helped during the early part of the trip, but about the time I was ready to fly home, my eyes were nearly swollen shut. The first thing I did when I got back to Oklahoma was to go to a doctor. Before I could tell him about my troubles, he observed that I had about the worst case of skin allergy he had ever seen. I told him how ineffective my antihistamines had been. He asked how much of my body was so affected and, after an examination of my itching body, remarked: "Cortisone is to be used in allergy cases only in emergencies. If this isn't an emergency, I never saw one. This prescription calls for 16 tablets. Take four a day and you should be over your skin condition in four days. The tablets will cost you fifty cents each. Go right ahead with your antihistamines; there will be no conflict with the cortisone."

At the end of the four days, my skin allergy was gone and I felt great. I said, "This is it; it's expensive, but it's worth it to stop these allergic attacks." I had at last found the end of the rainbow for which I had been looking for so many years. My enthusiasm for my new remedy, cortisone, was short-lived, however, for I soon learned from the doctors that the cure was worse than the disease.

At last I had definitely established to my satisfaction that one hormone from the adrenal glands, cortisone, could and would put an end to a severe allergic attack when everything else had failed. Where I went from there I had not the slightest idea, but I had the feeling I wasn't far from the cure for allergies. How right I was!

6. In 1958, I inadvertently overlooked paying a disability premium on a United States government life insurance policy. The disability clause provided that after I became 65 no more premiums would be required. As soon as they received my application for reinstatement, the Veterans Administration wrote me that since only one more annual premium would be due on the disability clause, I would have to go to a Veterans Administration hospital for a physical examination. A day for the examination was suggested, which I immediately accepted.

At this hospital I was given a fairly thorough examination. One of the doctors stated to me: "Your blood pressure is way too low. Have you ever been treated for Addison's disease?" I informed him I had not, and I then asked: "Doctor, what is the significance of my low blood pressure?" He remarked that low blood pressure readings were usually indicative of decreased chemical activity within the body. "In your case," he said, "I would imagine the adrenal glands are involved."

In March, 1959, Dr. J. Wendall Mercer, our family physician and a general practitioner, put me on the diet and medication for hypoadrenocorticism. I can truthfully say I enjoyed the diet from the first day, and the only complaint I had was about the headaches I suffered after I eliminated coffee. When one has been a heavy coffee drinker for 50 years, he should not expect to get over the effects of the caffeine immediately. It was about two weeks before I adjusted to being without coffee.

For one week, I had an adrenal cortex extract injection each day. For the next three weeks, I got the shots three times each week, and then, for about three months, twice each week. After that, I got only a shot each week until the end of nine months, at which time I got a shot every other week until the end of one year, or March, 1960.

At that time, I told Dr. Mercer I believed I was cured and would discontinue the injections and the diet. He advised against doing so. His statement was: "You had allergies a long time before you started this program. You admit you like the diet, and you have never had a sore arm from the injections. Why don't you continue for another year? You have had most of your expense this first year. We will try giving you the shots every four weeks and see how you get along." I have not taken adrenal cortex extract since 1961.

After I had good health and my previous symptoms of allergy had been alleviated, I discussed my case with four doctors, all friends of mine. None of them had ever treated me, and their reactions to my enthusiastic report of what had happened were most pessimistic.

Dr. A. said he would not want a patient of his to have "all that steroid injected into his body."

Dr. B. responded by saying: "You patients build up a lot of psychological momentum over something new and fantastic, but it won't last."

Dr. C. stated his patients couldn't afford such luxurious foods and drugs.

Dr. D. indicated he would go along with those specially trained in allergies until they changed their minds about what methods they would use.

Why did all four of these excellent physicians take such a defensive attitude? I had not accused them of doing anything wrong. Was it because I, a layman, may have expressed a medical opinion? Was it because they believed a layman is always wrong in his opinions about his own physical condition? It couldn't be because doctors are always right. As a trial judge, I have gotten so used to hearing certain doctors testify for complainants in damage suits and certain other well-known insurance company doctors testify for the parties sued, that I frequently know in advance, from reading the pleadings in the cases, approximately what each doctor is going to tell the court and jury.

It is easy for me to understand the doctors' conservatism because I belong to a profession that is more conservative than theirs. Lawyers generally are opposed to any changes in practice or procedure. They remind me of the old man who lived 50 years on the farm his father homesteaded 100 years before. A tourist stopped at the farm to make some inquiry and, after learning how long the man had resided there, remarked, "You must have seen many changes in your nation, state, and community in the past 50 years." The old gentleman answered, "Yes, I have; and I have been against all of them."

It is only natural that some physicians express opposition to any plan of treating allergies different from the one employed by the allergists a half century. Even if every patient who received the adrenal cortex extract and followed the anti-hypoglycemia diet were to experience complete recovery from all allergic diseases, some reactionary doctors would brand the method of treatment as unorthodox, unconventional and unsafe until more was known about it. I read somewhere that penicillin was not accepted generally by the medical profession until nearly twenty-five years after it was discovered.

The important thing to keep in mind is that there are no records of any patient having suffered any adverse effects from the use of the whole adrenal cortex extract. Those doctors who have not approved this method of treating allergies do not contend it can or will have any harmful effect. Their objections are based on grounds other than injury to a patient. We should remember that adrenal cortical extracts were used and considered harmless by physicians who prescribed them long before cortisone or other steroids were available.

Returning to the objections of some doctors to the hypoadrenocorticism treatment of allergies, let us examine their principal objections and see how much merit, if any, there is in what they say.

1. Some of my inquirers have reported back to me that their doctors said the treatment was one generally accepted by the medical profession. To make such a statement is, of course, to say the obvious. I dare say nearly every routine treatment employed daily in a doctor's office was not, at one time, generally accepted by the medical profession. We don't have to confine our remarks to medicine to know that most of our everyday actions haven't always been accepted as the most effective way of doing things. This objection, if we dignify it by calling it that, is too absurd to discuss further.

2. A few doctors, so I hear, claim adrenal cortex extract has only "historical value," whatever that means. These doubting Thomases should read the medical histories of thousands upon thousands of allergics, who, after trying everything recommended to them by their doctors, despaired of ever having good health until they found this new and phenomenal way to relief. These histories will provide something of "historical value" to the medical profession now and in the years to come.

If we assume these doctors mean that proponents of the adrenocorticism method of treatment must produce statistics showing how many dogs, cats, rabbits, mice, and the like have responded favorably to adrenal cortex extract in allergy cases, their position is preposterous. As Dr. E. M. Abrahamson so aptly pointed out, man is the only animal known to suffer from allergies.

These "historical value" physicians daily prescribe

cortisone, ACTH, and other steroid compounds, knowing the danger that can and will result therefrom. They know that adrenal cortex extract will never cause any bad side effects.

3. Some doctors bitterly object to the term "subclinical Addison's disease" used by physicians who have had close to one hundred percent success in the treatment of chronic allergy cases — patients who had been discarded by reputable physicians and frequently found their way into the clutches of unscrupulous practitioners before they were told about the new way of curing allergies.

To the layman's way of thinking, it makes no difference whether these people were or were not suffering from "subclinical Addison's disease." The only thing of importance to the patient is that he got relief from his suffering. I go along with the doctors who call the condition of these distressed people "subclinical Addison's disease" solely because they were right and other doctors were wrong in alleviating my symptoms.

4. Physicians have objected to the cost of the treatments. It is true that the adrenal cortex extract is expensive, and a high protein diet costs more than one loaded with bread, potatoes, rice, and pies or cakes.

It would seem that the patients instead of the doctors should be the ones to complain about costs. Over a long period of years, an allergic patient will spend a lot of money for medical and drug bills and still be seeking relief. If the patient recovers his health, or improves it by means of diet and medication, the medical and food expenses may well be, in the long run, the cheapest medication and food costs the patient ever had.

Before a doctor becomes too upset about what his patient is going to have to spend for food and adrenal cortex extract, I suggest he turn the picture around and have a look at what he may see on the other side. I am talking about a young or middle-aged wage earner whose only source of income is what he makes with his head and his hands, a worker with excellent earning capacity, but unable to keep a good job because of lack of health. Is that treatment too expensive for such a person? Should he be disposed of by having his cards at the employment agencies marked "Irascible and undesirable," or should he be given treatments, even if expensive? This man is not looking for hand-outs for himself and his family. Almost every one of these people has a sense of dignity and a respect for the rights and properties of others, regardless of how poverty stricken he may have become as a result of his inability to get and hold a job because of his allergic diseases.

Do I consider my recovery too expensive? I'll let you be the judge of that. The entire cost to me of the adrenal cortex therapy was less than the average cost in 1959 or 1960 of one major operation performed every day in practically every hospital in the nation. My proof for this statement came from figures released by national and state hospital associations.

As I shall later show, there are innumerable ways to lower the cost of a high protein diet. We live well, and our grocery bills are no higher than those of our friends whose incomes are comparable to ours. Regardless of how much some doctors may want to sympathize with me about the cost of adrenal cortex extract and good food, I can't put a price tag on the value of good health.

In the damage suits brought to my courts, juries and I, as the trial judge, try to determine in dollars the value of good health to one who has lost it by the negligence of another. What is the monetary value of good health? Would you say ten thousand dollars, twenty-five thousand dollars, a hundred thousand dollars, or even more?

While some doctor is fuming about the high cost of adrenal cortex extract and high protein foods, another doctor — maybe the family physician who helped bring the patient or his children into the world — is getting tremendous pleasure from helping his patient regain health and strength and take his rightful place in society. Which of these physicians do you believe is the wiser?

6.

A DIET YOU WILL LIKE

I know that most people, especially men, object to any kind of diet. I also know that many women have unsuccessfully been on a myriad of diets, trying to get back their youthful figures. Nearly all articles on reducing either start or conclude with the statement that obese persons eat more than their bodies require; that reduction of daily caloric consumption is the only way to reduce. Short term crash diets are starvation diets. Prepared liquid reducing foods are generally too high in carbohydrates to have much reducing value.

Calories do count when it comes to gaining or losing weight. Measuring and weighing every food item to get a certain number of calories is distasteful to most of us. The antihypoglycemia diet is low in calories, high in nutritional value, and can readily be adjusted to your bodily needs. I can take off weight easily and quickly by cutting down on my carbohydrates; that I have never eaten less protein and salad foods while reducing, accounts for my never having been abnormally hungry since I started the diet in 1959.

Once you get your weight where you want it, you can start increasing some carbohydrate foods. You will soon find how easy it is to keep your weight the same without that half-starved feeling with which you are so familiar.

A disadvantage of starvation diets is that one who has been on one of them looks older after he has lost weight. If you follow the antihypoglycemia diet, however, you will look younger as the pounds melt away.

Please do not get the impression that this diet was worked out for weight reducers. It is aimed at improving the function of the endocrines — particularly the adrenals and the pancreas, with its islands of Langerhans. However, it is a wonderful reducing diet.

One benefit of the diet and the adrenal cortex medication is that they slow down the course of degenerative diseases that normally come with the years, arteriosclerosis and many others. My own experience with the diet convinced me that getting old is largely the result of malnutrition. Doctors tell us that most people who have aged prematurely have been starved of vitamins and minerals. Often, these doctors say, it is difficult to pinpoint the direct cause of malnutrition since the subjects are subclinical cases rather than the classical textbook examples of malnutrition.

Medical science has a long way to go in the field of biochemistry. Dr. Sam E. Roberts said, in his book, *Ear, Nose and Throat Dysfunctions Due to Deficiencies and Imbalances:* "The medical students of the past who are our physicians today were taught little or nothing of nutrition and even less of deficiencies and imbalances. The authors of of *Therapeutic Nutrition* remark that medical school curricula are preoccupied with diagnosis and specific therapy. Little time and attention is given to the nutritional aspect of therapeutics." Dr. Roberts went on to point out that although biochemistry is taught today, it is taught without any clinical application or understanding. Dr. Roberts' views were approved in a foreword to the book by Dr. Morris Fishbein, whose name is a household word in American medicine.

Dr. Charles E. Butterworth, Jr., chairman of the American Medical Association's Council on Food and Nutrition, wrote in the March-April, 1974, issue of *Nutrition Today* that hospital physicians who are marvelously adept at performing the latest surgical procedures are so ignorant or lackadaisical about basic nutrition that their patients needlessly suffer complications, poor healing, extended recoveries, and even outright starvation leading to death. After reviewing many case histories, Dr. Butterworth said the astounding ignorance of physicians is only the logical result of the "long standing neglect of nutrition in medical education and in health care delivery systems."

Dr. David Baird Cousin said in the November, 1974, *American Journal of Clinical Nutrition*: " . . . few medical schools have a continuously comprehensive teaching program in the field . . . of nutrition."

Dr. Ross Hall, professor of biochemistry at McMaster University medical school, Hamilton, Ontario, concluded in the January 2, 1975, British magazine,

New Scientist, that nutrition is not only stagnating but "is still in the 19th century." The shocking thing about this great Canadian physician's article is the apparent ignorance of physicians in 1975 regarding vitamin deficiencies and their relation to clinical diseases.

An editorial in the British medical journal, *The Lancet,* October 26, 1974, had this to say: "If a fraction of the attention devoted to assessing new drugs was turned on to diets, it could reap handsome rewards for the science of therapeutics."

You may be a little frightened at the prospect of having foods to which you are accustomed eliminated from your diet, but there is no occasion for alarm. It did not take me long to turn my attention from the bakeries and sweet shops to the dietetic counters and low calorie sections of grocery stores and supermarkets. You will be surprised at what you find in these stores. The artificially sweetened syrups, jellies, and preserves are as tasty as those you have been eating. Every kind of canned fruit is available without sugar. The diet includes nearly all fresh fruits, and only a few vegetables are not permitted.

When fresh fruit is not available, I buy water-packed fruit in gallon cans and sweeten it with artificial sweeteners. Unsweetened canned fruits do not cost as much as those to which sugar has been added. Every nutritional expert says that low priced meats have as much nutritional value as high priced cuts.

Occasionally you may eat a small waffle or hot cake made from gluten and/or soybean flour, using, of course, artificially sweetened syrup or jelly. At one time I made a list of over 100 different desserts which could be included on the diet. If one feels he must eat ice cream, he may have small servings of dietetic (sugarless) ice cream. The low-calorie gelatin desserts which are prepared without sugar are delicious and inexpensive, and sugarless bottled or canned soft drinks are as good and about the same price as sweetened soft drinks. Each morning I look forward to two cups of decaffeinated coffee with as much enthusiasm as I formerly had for regular coffee.

There are many things we should keep in mind about why we are on this diet and what we hope to accomplish with it. We take snacks between meals and before bedtime, when it is necessary to keep our blood sugar from falling. If we eat three fairly good meals and no more during a day there will be three upward and three downward swings of the blood sugar level, but if we eat less at meal times, and oftener, then were will be six or seven up and down swings.

When we eat sugar, candy, honey, ice cream, pie, cake, or any quickly absorbed carbohydrates, the sudden rise in blood sugar level stimulates the islets of the pancreas to produce more insulin. The insulin, in turn, gets rid of too much blood sugar and lowers the blood sugar level. This sudden drop is what makes us feel so terrible, and generally starts some kind of allergic attack. An emotional upset also causes the islets of the pancreas to produce more insulin. Therefore, we only eat carbohydrates that are absorbed slowly, and we avoid any stress that causes a sudden drop in blood sugar level. You may have no more breakfasts of coffee and doughnuts or sweet rolls while on this diet.

There are many ways the cost of the diet may be

kept down. Instant nonfat powdered milk is cheaper than regular milk and just as nutritious. You can eliminate milk and take plain bone meal tablets at a cost of only a few cents a day. Nutritional experts generally recommend that a patient should not drink more than one quart of milk daily to avoid the danger of developing calcium stones in the kidney or bladder. If cheese or cream is used, the milk supply should be reduced accordingly. A pint of milk a day, or its equivalent in other calcium and phosphorus foods, is ordinarily adequate for an adult.

Doctors recommend · increasing the amount of water intake in order to prevent the formation of calcium stones. They tell us that normally our kidneys excrete any excess of blood calcium if we have an adequate supply of liquids daily.

We should remember that we eat foods to furnish the materials for growth and repair, to provide energy for our work and the functional activities of the organs and tissues of the body, and to maintain body temperature. There is no hard and fast rule as to what part of your diet should be carbohydrate and what part protein.

An inverse ratio exists throughout the world between carbohydrate consumption and income. In America, carbohydrates are normally expected to meet roughly 50 per cent of the total energy requirements. In the tropics and in some impoverished parts of the world, carbohydrates contribute up to 80 per cent of the daily caloric needs.

Roughly speaking, carbohydrates should not furnish more than one third of the hypoglycemic's daily caloric energy. Enough fat must be taken to supply the essential fatty acids and fat soluble vitamins. The diet will always provide a sufficient amount of proteins for the work of the defense mechanisms, for tissue repair and maintenance, and for growth, since there is practically no limit on the protein foods allowed.

We must not forget that protein and fat supply potential glucose, which is made available very gradually through metabolic processes. It is best to have our largest protein meal in the evening. Although breakfast is the most important meal of the day, it is essential to have a high protein meal in the evening, since the glucose produced gradually from the protein foods is instrumental in preventing hypoglycemia at night or early in the morning. If we eat an evening meal of quickly absorbed carbohydrates, insulin destroys so much of our blood sugar by or before midnight that we have headaches and an "all in" feeling, and we develop hay fever, asthma, or some other allergic symptom by morning.

Whenever I eat a large steak for dinner, I always take a bedtime snack of some slowly absorbed carbohydrate food (generally fruit) to prevent insulin induced hypoglycemia during the night.

Most of us grew up with the belief that we had to eat some sugar every day. This view still persists with many people even though the theory that we need sugar in our diets was exploded years ago. More and more doctors are coming to the conclusion that nobody needs sugar, although persons with normal blood sugar generally are able to eat a reasonable amount of sugar with no harmful effects.

Saccharin and other sugar substitutes have long

been uses by diabetics and are usually harmless. They are inexpensive compounds and have no calories, and you will find them as delicious as cane or beet sugar. Some persons, however, have told me tht they are allergic to one or more of the artificial sweeteners and that they break out in a skin rash or skin irritation after a long period of use. I don't believe this is a common complaint of users of saccharin or other sugar substitutes, but if an allergy should appear, it would be advisable to discontinue use until you determine whether the sweetener is the cause of the allergic condition.

There are three fallacies about older people you should know:

1. *As one grows older, he should become heavier.* Most older persons gain weight as the years pass, although it was not nature's intention. We overeat, eat the wrong kinds of foods, and don't exercise enough. Weight should not increase with the years. The insurance companies' physicians say we should weigh approximately the same at 26 and 62.

2. *We should discontinue exercising as we grow older.* Of course an inactive old man or old woman should not go out and do some violent exercising that will bring on a heart attack. Physicians generally agree, however, that there is as much need for a 70-year-old person to take some reasonable exercise each day if he is to remain strong and healthy, as there is for a ten-year-old child to run and play.

3. *Older people should not eat much.* There is no difference in the mineral and vitamin requirements of the young and the old. The bones of many older people are very fragile. Formerly, doctors thought

that demineralization of the bones was caused by a low calcium diet, but now they are confident that it is the result of several additional factors, such as (1) reduced secretion of hormones, (2) reduced absorption of food through the intestines due to malabsorption, (3) reduced intake of vitamin D, and, for the most part, (4) an inadequate protein diet. Many older people are strongly prejudiced against drinking milk and eating foods high in protein content.

The generally accepted diet for those in their later years is one high in proteins, rich in vitamins and minerals, moderately low in carbohydrates, and low in fats. Oldsters should be required to drink a generous amount of liquids throughout the day — water, milk, coffee and tea when permitted, and fruit juices.

Our older citizens do not look on changes with much favor. Changes usually have to come gradually and with some carefully planned persuasion. When an old man or woman refuses to drink milk, the easiest way to introduce minerals into the diet is by mixing dried nonfat milk in a soup or other food at meal time. If milk in any form is refused, the person may be prevailed upon to take bone meal tablets. Sometimes it really takes a diplomat to get an old man or an old woman to accept the foods he or she should eat.

One of the comparatively new developments in food technology is the enrichment and fortification of refined or compounded and processed foods with specific minerals or vitamins. Enrichment and fortification has become accepted routine procedure in the preparation of many popular foods.

Also, since World War II, many foods have been

dehydrated to prevent spoilage; the process is safe and involves little or no loss in vitamins and minerals. Persons who cannot eat the fresh products can sometimes tolerate dried milk and dried eggs. Canning, freezing and refrigeration are other major methods of food preservation. Fruits and vegetables canned within 24 hours of picking have higher vitamin content than fresh fruits and vegetables bought on the open market after prolonged shipping and storage.

Glycogen (the form in which the liver stores carbohydrates) is also found in small quantities in practically all other organs of the body. The skeletal, cardiac, and smooth muscles maintain their own glycogen stores when at rest or under minor work loads. The conversion of glucose into glycogen is reversible; when quick absorption of carbohydrates (especially glucose) raises the blood sugar level, the tide is counteracted by glycogenesis in the liver and withdrawal of glucose from circulation by body tissues for the purposes of energy metabolism and storage against future needs. Glycogenesis has been defined as the conversion of glycogen into glucose or the conversion of glucose into glycogen. (See Webster's International Dictionary and Stedman's Medical Dictionary.)

Despite the continual danger warnings in the newspapers, magazines, and other news media, more than 20 per cent of all adults are overweight to the extent that health may be impaired. We are told that obesity aggravates cardiovascular disease and osteoarthritis. It may cause hypertension, atherosclerosis, hernia, and gallbladder disease. In predisposed persons, it may bring on diabetes. It makes surgery more hazardous, causes postural derangement, and makes a person appear older than he actually is. Mortality from most diseases is much higher among the obese.

Unfortunately, the obese have been victimized by many products advertised as harmless weight reducers. All sorts of pharmaceutical preparations are available and sometimes sold without prescriptions. These include appetite depressants, substances which increase the basal metabolism rate, and metabolized vegetable gums. Few physicians regard these as desirable aids in reducing weight.

When I started the diet and the medication in 1959, I had one purpose in mind — to alleviate my allergic diseases. When I discovered that the diet was wonderful for reducing and obtaining good health, you can understand how jubilant I was. My enthusiasm for and my belief in the antihypoglycemia diet are unbounded. With this diet one may achieve what he dreams about, but never expects to experience — he may find relief from allergic diseases, regain good health, return to a trim and youthful figure, attain emotional stability, and slow down the degenerative diseases that go with age.

If your tests and physical examination indicate that this new plan for overcoming allergies might help you, all I ask is that you give it a fair and reasonable trial. It won't be long before you can tell whether it will do for you what it did for me. If it doesn't work with you after a reasonable time, drop it. No harm will have been done and it won't be the first money you have spent on something recommended to you without beneficial results.

If and when you go on the diet, use your imagination and curiosity in selecting your meals and snacks. There is no more reason for you to be bored by monotony than there was before you started the treatment. There are so many, many foods you are permitted to eat.

I repeat, it is imperative that you stay on the diet every day. If you eat out, you will have no difficulties, since restaurants will gladly make substitutions for the starchy vegetables that come with regular meals. Most waitresses will assume that you are a diabetic and do their best to obtain foods you can eat. Cafeterias will be your best bet for getting what you want and may eat.

The practice of saying No to offers of coffee, sweets, and other forbidden foods when you attend parties, committee meetings, teas, after-meeting refreshment periods and the like, will become a valuable habit when rich desserts are offered you, even after you leave the diet.

The diet will appeal to women because they are natural shoppers. I have always hated shopping, but I enjoy going through grocery stores, supermarkets, department stores, drug stores, and health food stores, looking for sugar-free and low carbohydrate foods, which I find in abundance. If you are not accustomed to so doing, you will soon learn to read what is on the printed labels of canned foods to find out the sugar and other carbohydrate contents.

SUGGESTED INEXPENSIVE MENU

On arising in the morning

Fruit juice not sweetened with sugar

Breakfast

One thin slice toasted protein bread with
butter or margarine and dietetic jelly
Fresh fruit or canned fruit artificially
sweetened
One egg; boiled, poached, scrambled or fried
Decaffeinated coffee

Mid-morning snack

Cheese (any kind) with 2 or 3 saltines

Lunch

Egg and cheese sandwich (open face) made with one
slice of toasted protein bread; butter or
margarine (not corn) optional
Sliced tomatoes
Serving of cooked vegetable
Molded gelatin dessert with or without artificially
sweetened mixed fruits
Milk or bone meal tablets

Mid-afternoon snack

Salted nuts or dietetic peanut butter rolled up
in a leaf of lettuce

Dinner

Mixed green vegetable with small amount of no-
sugar French or mayonnaise dressing

Hamburger steak
Serving of cooked vegetable
Any permitted fruit for dessert
Decaffeinated coffee

Bedtime snack

Glass of milk and one thin slice of protein bread
or 2 or 3 saltines

SUGGESTED MENU — MORE EXPENSIVE

On arising in the morning

Fruit juice not sweetened with sugar

Breakfast

Ham or sausage and one egg
One thin slice protein bread, toasted if desired,
with butter or margarine
Fruit, such as half grapefruit, orange, non-
sweetened apple sauce, or any other fruit
not excluded from diet
Decaffeinated coffee

Mid-morning snack

Milk or dietetic peanut butter and 2 or 3 saltines

Lunch

Grated carrot and cabbage or lettuce salad
Chicken or fish
Cooked vegetable

One slice of protein bread (toasted if desired)
with butter or margarine
Melon, any kind

Mid-afternoon snack

Salted nuts

Dinner

Cottage cheese salad
Pork chops or lamb chops
Cooked vegetable
Cooked dried fruit or fresh fruit
Decaffeinated coffee

Bedtime snack

Glass of milk and some permitted fruit

SUGGESTED MENU — MORE EXPENSIVE

On arising in the morning

Fruit juice not sweetened with sugar
Breakfast

Bacon and two eggs
One thin slice protein bread (may be toasted)
with butter or margarine and artificially
sweetened fruit preserves
Half grapefruit, half cantaloupe, or any kind
of permitted fruit
Decaffeinated coffee

Mid-morning snack

Glass of milk and 2 or 3 saltines

Lunch

Cottage cheese salad with avocado or
unsweetened pineapple
Ham, ground steak, fish, or fowl
One cooked vegetable
One slice of protein bread (toasted if desired)
with butter or margarine

Mid-afternoon snack

Salted nuts

Dinner

Tossed green salad with or without small amount of
no-sugar French or mayonnaise dressing
Roast beef or steak, latter preferably broiled
One cooked vegetable
Dietetic ice cream
Decaffeinated coffee

Bedtime snack

Glass of milk with thin slice of protein bread or
dietetic peanut butter and 2 or 3 saltines

THINGS TO REMEMBER ABOUT YOUR DIET

Milk

Children up to 12 years old need at least a pint of milk daily, and adolescents need at least 1 1/2 pints of milk daily. Adults generally need a pint of milk daily, but there are some adults who do not need and cannot digest that much. If other mineral products are served, the amount of milk may be reduced: 1 1/2 ounces of regular cheese or 2 or 3 scoops of dietetic (sugarless) ice cream count as a cup of milk. Raw, pasteurized, canned, or powered milk all have about the same food value.

Water

Drink lots of water. I suggest you drink the equivalent of 6 or 8 glasses of water (1 1/2 to 2 quarts) daily. Other fluids — such as decaffeinated coffee, milk, or fruit juice — may be counted in the amount of liquid suggested above.

Vitamins

Vitamins (whether taken in foods or as vitamin supplements) are foods, not medicines. Vitamins A and D, if taken in excess, can be toxic and may cause insomnia, headaches, restlessness, and irritability. Unless taken over a prolonged length of time and in exorbitant amounts, the toxic condition caused by excessive vitamin supplements generally disappears after use is discontinued. Remember, we get vitamin D from the sun, and some of our foods are enriched and fortified with additional vitamins. Taking excessive amounts of citrus fruits and their juices over a long period of time may produce an alkalized system, indicated by nasal itching and sometimes by small fissures in the nose, as well as by headaches, restlessness, and inability to sleep. This condition may be corrected by temporarily discontinuing the use of ascorbic acid foods and by the temporary administration of hydrochloric acid by your doctor.

Meats, Fish, and Poultry

One can, of course, overdo anything, but on this diet you are expected to eat meats, fish and poultry. I recommend that you eat liver frequently. You should eat eggs at least three times a week. If your physician has you on a low cholesterol diet, you must follow his recommendations about all cholesterol foods, including eggs, and disregard anything stated here to the contrary.

Mid-meal and Bedtime Snacks

Keep in mind always that your purpose in eating these snacks is to keep your blood sugar level as stable as possible. You are not to have six or seven meals a day, only three, and your regular meals are to be smaller because of your snacks. I have eaten almost every kind of food at snack time. The ones I have enjoyed most are fresh fruits, salted nuts, cheeses, peanut butter, milk, dietetic ice cream, beans, dietetic candies, and bits of fresh vegetables. At first you may be inclined to overdo on the snacks, but you will soon learn the proper amounts you should eat. After you have been on the diet a month or so, you may find you do not need to snack and that your three daily meals supply all the food you need.

If you think of your diet as the beginning of a wonderful new experience in the field of nutrition and health, rather than a boring something to be tolerated for a year or so, I am sure you will find it rewarding and enjoyable. It was part of the gateway to a new life for me, and I hope you will find it as fascinating and profitable as I did.

Plan your meals and then enjoy them. Meal patterns vary in various parts of the United States and at various seasons of the year. Before 1959, I ate meals from a sense of duty — generally eating too fast and paying either little or no attention to what I ate, mostly wondering whether I was eating foods to which I was allergic. Now, I like to take an hour or more to eat a seafood dinner or an Oklahoma steak, and find as much pleasure in so doing as I do when I see two of the nation's leading college football teams play or when I sit in the grandstand watching a close major league baseball game.

7.

VITAMINS AND ENZYMES

Much has been written about the body's daily vitamin requirements. Most physicians take the view that a well balanced diet contains most, if not all, of the essential vitamins. Nearly all doctors are of the opinion that there are times when certain vitamin supplements should be prescribed for some patients. Taking vitamins indiscriminately for any and all diseases, however, is looked upon with disfavor by the medical profession.

I am not inclined to start an argument with my medical friends about vitamins, but I believe their assumption that a well balanced diet furnishes all of the needed vitamins overlooks one question: "How many people have a well balanced diet daily?" What I know about the most common eating habits and what I have learned from my studies in nutrition have convinced me that few people have a well balanced diet.

Just as money is wasted on some unnecessary vitamin supplements, so is it wasted on erroneously prescribed medicines. Nevertheless, it would be ridiculous for me to say that I am not going to call a doctor when I become ill because my hypoglycemic condition was not correctly diagnosed until 1959. There is no doubt in my mind that for the remainder of my life I will take vitamin A, B, C, D and E supplements.

In my opinion, some vitamins are more closely related to allergies than others. I have already talked about pantothenic acid, and I want to tell you about my experiences with vitamin E.

This vitamin has been one of the most controversial subjects in medicine in the United States. Most doctors contend that we get a sufficient amount of vitamin E in our normal diet, whereas other American doctors, certainly in the minority, take the view that many patients need to take supplements of vitamin E daily. There have been reports of improvement and cure of diseases of the cardiovascular system from the addition of vitamin E to the diet. Other doctors have scoffed at such claims as being fantastic and unreasonable and have asserted that vitamin E could not have played such a role.

Doctors in Canada and Europe generally have a more positive attitude to the use of vitamin E supplements in treating specific diseases than have American physicians. I accidentally came across some Canadian medical publications which stated, in substance, that vitamin E plays an important role physiologically in inhibiting or reducing the tendency of oxygen to combine with other substances and produce a toxic condition. Stated another way, they asserted that with many people oxygen combines with other elements to form toxic compounds and that vitamin E is an antioxidant. One article stated that because of this reductioñ-oxidation property, vitamin E is important in the end stages of carbohydrate metabolism.

These articles intrigued me for several reasons. I asked myself these questions: (1) Is it possible that a lack of vitamin E caused me to have breathing difficulties? (2) Were the nasal (rhinitis) attacks which followed the eating of certain foods at least partially caused by a toxic compound resulting from oxygen combining with some substance or substances in the offending food? (3) In case the answer to question 2 is Yes, would vitamin E supplement inhibit the formation of the toxic compound? (4) Was it possible that the "oxygen-combining" theory of these Canadian physicians was more correct than the "allergen sensitivity" theory of most American doctors?

The only way I knew to get the answer to these questions was to experiment with vitamin E. In 1956 I secured a large bottle of the most potent vitamin E capsules available. I started taking 1000 or more units daily and soon experienced all kinds of difficulties. I didn't sleep well, I was more nervous than usual, my allergies worsened and I had a dull headache most of the time. After a few weeks, I gave up the vitamin E experiment, threw away the remaining capsules and decided anyone who tried to be his own doctor had a fool for a patient.

Early in 1960, while I was making remarkable progress with the antihypoglycemia diet and medication, I came across another medical article about vitamin E. My first inclination was not to read it. I was certain I had read enough medical quackery about vitamin E to last a lifetime. Curiosity was too much, so I read the article. It stated that a patient going on vitamin E should never start with more than 100 units daily as the vitamin in larger amounts has a tendency at first to raise blood pressure and cause the symptoms I experienced from 1000 units a day.

For nearly a month I weighed the pros and cons of again trying vitamin E supplementation. One day I bought a bottle of vitamin E and for about ten days I took 100 units daily. Nothing of importance happened. I then started taking 600 units each day and the effect of the vitamins was phenomenal. My nasal passages opened as they had done when I took astringent nasal drops and my hearing improved as my nose and throat cleared up. Instead of using only the upper part of my lungs to breathe, I seemed to be using all of my lungs.

Physicians from every state and many foreign countries have told me their allergic patients had similar experiences to mine after experimenting with vitamin E.

Now that physicians have discovered that hypo-glycemics (low blood sugar sufferers) have nearly a two to one chance over those with normal blood sugar of death from vascular (blood vessel) disease, and that diabetics (high blood sugar sufferers) have an even higher rate of death from circulatory disease, we can take a look at recent medical literature and see why vitamin E is so important to all with abnorm-al blood sugar conditions.

Drs. E. Cheraskin and W. M. Ringsdorf, Jr., of the University of Alabama, reported on vitamin E in the August, 1970, issue of *Nutrition Report International.* They gave these startling facts: "The data confirm with the well-established fact that with advancing age there are progressively more cardiovascular symptoms and signs . . . Cardiovascular findings do increase with age, but only in those subjects consuming suboptimal amounts of vitamin E."

Other physicians have recently told us that if we eat polyunsaturated fats we must take vitamin E supplements as antioxidants to prevent ischemia, (deficiency. of blood due to constrictions of the blood vessels) and cancer.

Medical articles are legion showing that heart sufferers plagued with the problem of insufficient oxygen have need for more vitamin E than is found in our usual meals.

Dr. L. M. Hursh of the University of Illinois, after warning that heated unsaturated fats strip the body of vitamin E stores, recently said: "There is one other problem no one ever discusses and that is the co-carcinogenic (cancerous) activity of heated unsaturated fat . . . This is a serious problem, but has gained little attention."

It should be observed that Germany has banned the reuse by reheating of polyunsaturated fats in commercial cooking.

Tests show that polyunsaturated fats in the body burn faster than do saturated fats, so we need vitamin E to maintain proper control of metabolism. This means that we, who eat polyunsaturated fats to prevent high cholesterol levels, should provide our bodies with more oxygen which comes from vitamin E.

Since vitamin E is slowly absorbed, the day's supply may be taken at one time, following a meal, preferably with some fat. Inorganic iron (the kind prescribed by doctors) destroys vitamin E in the body, so medicated iron should not be taken for 12 hours after taking supplementary vitamin E.

Many physicians believe there is some relationship between vitamin C and the production of the adrenal cortex hormones in view of the high concentration of this vitamin in the adrenals.

The discovery within the past few years that vitamin C, when taken often and in rather large amounts, acts as an antihistamine, *without any adverse side effects,* was great news to all allergics.

This vitamin is by far the most glamorous of all. Not a month goes by but the medical journals report some new discovery of the effectiveness of vitamin C in preventing or helping cure some disease.

We know that stress plays a big part in causing all allergic condition. A few weeks ago a surgeon chided me about my outspoken views favoring vitamin supplements. I asked him: "Why do you prescribe vitamin C before, during and after surgery?" His answer was: "To protect our patients against the stress resulting from surgery."

Another doctor said to me recently: "My wife has read your books and has been taking vitamin supplements. I hate to admit it, but her health has improved tremendously."

The most controversial of all vitamins is vitamin P, or the bioflavanoids. Branded as ineffective and worthless by the Food and Drug Administration, the bioflavanoids are being recommended by leading physicians to prevent, alleviate or cure allergies, glaucoma, peridontal disease and many others. I have found the vitamin effective in preventing bruises, especially on my hands, resulting from capillary fragility. Hundreds of doctors and laymen have told me how the formation of the red or purple spots, later turning brown, caused by little or no impact with objects, can be prevented by the bioflavanoids.

I found that oranges, when the outside covering is cut off with a sharp knife, leaving the white pulp, are very effective. I eat all of the peeled orange except the seed. The pulp and connecting tissue of the orange are where we find vitamin P, not in the juice, which is rich in vitamin C. This is also true of grapefruit and other citrus fruits. Rutin tablets are a good source of vitamin P.

You will find in medical literature that bioflavanoids have done these things:

1. Helped cure respiratory infections.
2. Lowered high blood pressure.
3. Stopped nose and gum bleeding.
4. Protected against radiation.
5. Been helpful in circulatory diseases.

Informed physicians have, for years, known that bioflavanoids prevent capillary weakness. One does not have to suffer a major stroke to experience the effects of weakness of these tiny blood vessels — the capillaries. If you have, for no apparent reason, had a sudden dizzy spell, had your arm or leg suddenly go weak, which you attribute to "clumsiness," or if you, without cause, while walking, apparently stumbled over something that was not there, you may have had a "little stroke" resulting from a failure of the blood supply to the brain.

Some of the other indicia of "little strokes" are mental confusion, loss of ability, lack of interest in life, premature aging and fear of being alone.

If you had a "little stroke," the chances are you never knew what it was and you may never suffer a major cerebral illness. It would be downright silly to worry continually about having a stroke. If you do have an experience that might be a "little stroke," you should immediately see your physician.

It only makes good sense to keep your capillaries strong by eating lots of fruits and vegetables high in vitamins C and P, and following the suggestions in a later chapter on heart attacks.

Unlike most of the lower animals, man does not manufacture or store vitamin C or vitamin P in the body. We must therefore be certain that we get a sufficient amount of these vitamins every day.

Physicians have determined that all B vitamins are important in helping promote the health of their patients suffering abnormal blood sugar levels. The B vitamins are essential to digestion and use of foods. Any plan that does not include good nutrition is shortsighted and not for the best interest of the allergic. Here are some medical opinions concerning B vitamins:

1. Dr. E. Cheraskin wrote in *The International Journal of Vitamin Research* (1967) that persons with heart complaints consumed the least amounts of thiamine, (vitamin B_1).

2. Dr. T. L. Kopjas in the November, 1966, *Journal of the American Geriatric Society*, reported that folic acid is an effective but harmless dilator of small blood vessels.

3. Dr. Henry Schroeder told us in the July, 1955, *Journal of Chronic Diseases* that pyridoxine (vitamin B_6) deficiency will cause hardening of the arteries and high blood pressure.

4. Dr. W. Stanley Hartroft wrote in the March, 1966, *American Journal of Public Health* that a choline deficient diet causes high blood pressure.

5. Dr. Louis B. Dotti and associates (see *Newsweek,* September 11, 1950) reported that another B vitamin, inositol, lowered cholesterol levels.

6. Many articles in medical journals have shown that niacin, another B vitamin, is effective in lowering cholesterol. Commenting on the failure of most physicians to show little interest in vitamins, Dr. William B. Parsons, Jr., suggested in *Medical Tribune,* (November 28, 1964) that if niacin could be patented, doctors might use it instead of drugs. Dr. Parsons said that drug companies, without the incentive to make large profits, aren't interested in promoting a cheap vitamin, as niacin, that can be bought over the counter without a prescription.

Dr. Miles Atkinson reported in *Archives of Otolarynogology* (1962) that migraine, an allergic disease, resulted from a vitamin B_3 (niacin) deficiency.

7. Dr. Hans Selye said in his book, *The Stress of Life,* that allergic symptoms are nothing more than the body's reaction to stress. Dr. T. Ogawa wrote in *The American Journal of Physiology* (1960) that pantothenic acid (a B vitamin) is as effective with allergy patients as steroid drugs.

In 1954 Iowa physicians gave volunteers from a state prison food deficient in pantothenic acid. During the second week these men became fatigued and had difficulty staying awake. By the fourth week they were quarrelsome, discontented and miserable. They developed low blood pressure, stomach disorders and respiratory infections. (See *Proceedings of the Society of Biology,* 1954).

We know how important pantothenic acid is to the proper functioning of the adrenal glands. When we consider the importance of all B vitamins in helping to lower body stress, it is not difficult to understand why our allergies are mostly nutrition in origin.

A few vitamins are synthesized in the intestines. Nutritionally educated physicians tell us that vitamins work best in combinations, for example, the danger of vitamin D being toxic is reduced by an adequate amount of vitamin A, and vitamin E is more effective as an antioxident when vitamin C is present in the body. These doctors have shown us how vitamins and minerals, working together, protect us from disease and increase our chances for long, healthy lives.

Enzymology is another branch of biochemistry, or the chemistry of life, about which even the experts have much to learn. Seventy years ago, enzymology was in its infancy as a branch of nutritional science concerned with the digestion of foods. It has grown in medical importance through the years, and we may now be on the threshold of discoveries that will give all of us a richer and fuller life and even provide the means for conquering and preventing most of the now-considered incurable diseases.

Enzymes control all of our body functions. We know much about vitamins and their importance to our health because vitamins have been glamorized by pharmaceutical-manufacturing companies for years. We know little about the 700 known enzymes without which vitamins would be worthless. In fact, many of the vitamins are coenzymes. As the *Columbia Health Bulletin* said in 1961: "They [enzymes] control man as they control all life, from the instant of conception to the moment he dies, his successes and failures, his characteristics and personality, his complete destiny."

You and I should be thankful that we live in the fabulous age of the study of enzymes. Scientists have barely entered this wonderful fairyland. What they will discover about these catalysts (substances having the power to cause other substances to produce chemical changes in living things) only time can tell. I hope I am among the living when many more of these secrets are revealed.

8.

YOU NEED THE MINERALS, TOO

The body needs about 13 different minerals, all of which must be obtained from the antihypoglycemia diet or from supplements. The minerals most likely to be present in our bodies in insufficient amounts are calcium, iron, magnesium, zinc and iodine. Ninety per cent of the body's ash consists of calcium and phosphorus. Ninety-nine per cent of the calcium and 80 per cent of the phosphorus are found in the skeletal tissues and teeth. None of the other required minerals even approaches one per cent of the total body composition.

Calcium

Absorption of dietary calcium takes place in the small intestine. Normal gastric hydrochloric acid and the presence of sufficient vitamin D facilitate the process.

Here in America where calcium intake is high because we use so much milk, cheese, ice cream and other dairy products, all bone-building foods, one would think that osteoporosis would be almost unknown. We likely have more middle-aged and older people with weak and fragile bones than has any other country. People in some other countries don't eat more than half as much calcium food as we eat.

Our doctors constantly boast that we are the best fed people in the world. Maybe we are are too well fed for our own good. We daily eat tremendous amounts of protein, especially beef.

Dr. Ralph Nelson of Mayos is quoted in the November 8, 1974, *Medical World News.* ". . . most people in this country eat perhaps twice as much protein as they need."

Helen Linkswiler and associates of the University of Wisconsin reported in April, 1974, issue of *Transactions of the New York Academy of Science* that with a moderate protein intake young male adults were in "calcium balance" whether their daily intake of calcium was 500 mg. or 1400 mg. These researchers found that with 47 grams of protein daily a moderate amount of 500 mg. of calcium was all that was needed. Yet we know that many adults consume 130 to 140 grams of protein (sometimes more) each day!

The medical experts say that large amounts of protein cause calcium to be washed out of the body in the urine. Medical researchers have known for a long time that adding meat to the diet increased the amount of calcium in the urine.

We were mistakenly told that protein promoted calcium absorption and the calcium in the urine was excessive and not needed. We were also unduly warned about the dangers of taking more than 400 units daily of vitamin D, which vitamin must be present in the body before calcium can be absorbed.

Before we decide what we are going to do about

changing our eating habits, lets see why a poorly absorbed and poorly utilized calcium supply may be dangerous to our health.

A constant supply of calcium is required in our bloodstream to build bones and control functions of the cells. If the calcium supply is below normal, the heartbeat becomes weaker and irregular. The body, trying to maintain a needed supply in the blood, borrows from the bones and returns the calcium when possible. We have know for a long time that calcium is essential to a regular and normal heartbeat.

Returning to the question of how much protein and how much calcium we need, the problem can be solved easily if we cut down on our meat supply and increase our supply of calcium and vitamin D.

Another reason we should lower our intake of meat, especially beef, is the increasing incidence of colon (lower bowel) cancer and the medical indications that it is the result of eating too much beef. Without going into detail, medical researchers have found that countries with a high intake of beef, saturated fat, sugar and white flour, have a high incidence of colon cancer, while those with lower beef and more high-fiber foods have less intestinal cancer.

Medical researchers have reasoned that the dietary fiber decreased stool transit time, increased moisture content of the stool and possibly acted directly on the intestinal flora.

Dr. E. W. Pomare of the British Royal Infirmary (*Internal Medicine News*, March 1, 1975) recommended the addition to our diet of completely unprocessed bran, the kind we find at health food stores, to avoid possible colon cancer.

You need protein in your diet. If you are a big meat eater, I suggest you eat less meat and more beans, grains, nuts and other vegetables high in protein. Fruits are always to be eaten. Unless you·are a heavy milk drinker, by all means take bone meal. Remember that four bone meal tablets ordinarily supply about 850 mg. of calcium. We should have about two and one half times as much calcium as phosphorus.

Within the past year medical researchers have given us some valuable information concerning osteoporosis in older people. They found that calcium bone loss *is reversible.* If your bones are not strong and fracture easily, you do not have to become a crippled old man or old woman. Your bone density will return, although *it will take time,* if you increase your calcium intake to somewhere between 1000 and 1500 mg. daily. You will be protecting your heart by so doing.

Your bones will be strengthened by exercise. When you walk or take other exercises, a weak electric current is generated which, in some unknown manner, draws calcium and other minerals out of the blood and into the bones, which are rebuilt and strengthened. That is the reason bones of athletes are so strong.

Don't get the mistaken and fatalistic attitude that you are "too old" to exercise. Your heartbeats are the result of muscular contraction caused by electric impulses. A brisk walk, when possible, at any age, is your best insurance that you will not become a "human vegetable" when you are old.

While you are eating bran and other bulk forming foods to prevent or control diverticulosis, don't overlook the fact that pantothenic acid aids in a more rapid transit of waste in the colon. If you drink lots of liquids, the unprocessed bran becomes soft and will not irritate your intestines.

If you have been taking tranquilizing drugs for nervousness, why not try additional calcium? Drs. Ferris Pitts, Jr., and James McClure, Jr., psychiatrists, presented a scientific study in the December 21, 1967, *New England Journal of Medicine,* showing that additional calcium overcomes anxiety neurosis.

Every year our medical researchers come up with some new and dramatic proof of the usefulness of calcium in preventing and curing disease.

Magnesium

Without going into detail, recent articles in the medical journals have shown that magnesium in our diet does these things:

1. With calcium, in proper proportion, it helps regulate the heartbeat.
2. It helps prevent high blood pressure.
3. It keeps us from having kidney stones.
4. It is essential to good heart health.
   This is accomplished, so we are told, by:
   [a] Lowering cholesterol in the bloodstream.
   [b] Overcoming the harmful effects of stress.
   [c] Not allowing deposits of calcium in the arteries.
   [d] Preventing hardening of the arteries.

Investigators have analyzed the mineral content of drinking water in many American cities and have always found a lower incidence of cardiovascular disease where the water is hard (high in magnesium) than in cities with soft water.

Phosphorus

This mineral has more body functions than any other. With calcium, it lends rigidity to the bones and teeth. About 80 per cent of the body's phosphorus is found in the skeletal tissue and teeth and the other 20 per cent is located in the body fluids and in every cell. Phosphorus metabolism is important in muscle-energy and nerve-tissue metabolism, in carbohydrate, protein, and fat metabolism, in normal blood chemistry, in skeletal growth and tooth development, as well as in the transport of fatty acids. It is also a component of many enzyme systems.

About 70 per cent of the phosphorus ingested is absorbed in the body. Vitamin D and a normal acid medium assist phosphorus absorption. The common foods which meet calcium and protein needs are usually simultaneously able to supply the required phosphorus.

The protein-rich foods — meat, fish, eggs and poultry — are excellent sources of this mineral. Milk, cheese, nuts and the legumes are also good sources of phosphorus.

Iron

This mineral plays an essential role in oxygen transport by the blood and in cellular respiration. It constitutes only .004 per cent of the body (4.5 grams in an average adult). Approximately one gram of this iron is stored in the liver and spleen.

Iron deficiency in man is one form of anemia, which may develop from inadequate diet or poor absorption. Blood loss, particularly chronic blood loss, may lead to anemia. Persons who harbor intestinal parasites or who suffer from bleeding hemorrhoids, bleeding ulcers, or recurrent nose bleeds are prone to iron deficiency.

The Food and Nutrition Board of the National Research Council recommends a daily intake of 10 to 15 milligrams of iron for adults and adolescents and 7 to 12 milligrams daily for children. These foods, in decreasing order of excellence, are good sources of iron: liver, heart, kidney, liver sausage, lean meats, shellfish, egg yolk, dried beans and other legumes, dried fruits, nuts, green leafy vegetables, whole grain and enriched cereals, and molasses. That milk is a poor source of iron accounts for the fact that infants must have foods containing iron to supplement milk.

Copper

The human diet usually supplies an adequate amount of copper. The daily minimum requirement of two milligrams of copper is supplied by even a poor diet. Copper is stored in the liver. Milk is low in copper, but a newborn baby has a stored-up liver supply of copper five to ten times greater than the supply of this mineral stored in an adult's liver. The best sources of copper are oysters, liver, beef, nuts, and mushrooms.

Iodine

This mineral is an essential nutrient since it plays such an important part in the formation of thyroid hormones, which regulate the metabolic rate. The output of the thyroid gland is affected by the availability of iodine. If the iodine supply is inadequate, the gland increases its secretory activity and enlarges until it becomes a goiter.

Iodine is absorbed from the small intestine. It is found in the blood as both inorganic iodine and protein-bound iodine. Optimal requirements for iodine in the adult range from .15 to .30 milligrams per day. Foods grown on iodine-poor soil contain insufficient iodine for meeting human needs. Goiter is frequently prevalent in those regions where there is a deficiency of iodine in the soil. They are sometimes call "goiter belts" or "goiter regions."

Among natural foods, the best sources of iodine are sea foods and vegetables grown on iodine-rich land, or kelp. The major source of iodine in America is iodized salt.

Cobalt

This mineral is known to compose about 4 per cent of vitamin B_{12}. It has been theorized that cobalt being so closely associated with vitamin B_{12}, may assist in preventing anemia. Cobalt is found in most foods and there is no known human requirement of the mineral. It has been speculated that cobalt may play a part in the normal metabolism of human growth.

Zinc

It was not until 1963 that the need for zinc in the human diet was discovered. In that short period of time we have learned that zinc supplementation does these things:

1. Promotes prostate health with men.
2. Hastens wound healing.
3. Helps bone formation.

4. Assists vitamin A absorption.

We are also told that zinc may:

[a] Be one of the nutrients whose deficiency causes epilepsy.

[b] Have anti-viral value.

[c] Be one of many elements deficient in the bodies of schizophrenics.

Studies are underway and have progressed far enough to strongly indicate that a deficiency of zinc in the diet may cause senility in older people.

A recent publication by some physicians in Israel (*The Complete Book of Minerals for Health*) by Goldman, et al., shows that the addition of zinc to the diet has a favorable effect on blood sugar levels. This suggests that zinc may play an important role in the proper functioning of the pancreases and in the metabolism of glucose for both hypoglycemics and diabetics.

Millions of dollars are spent each year advertising products that are claimed to prevent offensive body odors. I know that the zinc tablets I get at a health food store and take each day protect me from any offensive odors of the body.

The world's greatest researchers of zinc and its importance to health say they have not had sufficient time to find the answers to most of the questions now being considered.

Fluorine

This mineral is important since it is normally present in bones and teeth to prevent dental caries. Although it is found in many foods, we acquire most of our fluorine from drinking water. The average daily diet, including foods cooked in water, provides .25 to .32 milligrams of fluoride. During the period of tooth formation, the child's diet should contain an additional supplement of fluoride equal to about 1 mg. daily. Many dentists have applied a 2 per cent sodium fluoride solution directly to the teeth, especially of younger people, and have reported that it was effective in controlling dental caries.

Many cities and communities now add sodium fluoride to their water supplies in an effort to prevent dental caries among the young. Fluoridated water usually contains 1 ppm of fluorine. (It is claimed that water containing as much as 1.8 ppm of fluorine may produce mottling of the dental enamel.)

Sodium and Potassium

These minerals are discussed in Chapter 10.

Water

This mineral is second only to oxygen in maintaining life. Water is not only an essential nutrient, but the major component of the body as well. It is the body's vehicle for chemical transport and the medium in which practically all metabolic reactions involving other nutrients take place. The Food and Nutrition Board recommends, under conditions of moderate temperature and normal exercise, an intake of one milliliter of water for each calorie of food.

Other Mineral Elements

Sulfur, aluminum, silicon, manganese and bromide, while always present in the body, have not as yet been demonstrated to affect normal metabolism. Investigators may later show that these elements (although present in small quantities) as well as some others, play roles in metabolism, digestion, and mental processes not even contemplated at this time.

The British Medical Journal, *The Lancet,* pointed out on May 14, 1966, that practically nothing was then known about trace minerals in nutrition, and about everything was yet to be learned about them. The editorial predicted that knowledge of trace minerals will have an impact comparable to that of vitamins. The entire field of mineral nutritional knowledge is a virgin wilderness waiting to be explored, said *The Lancet.* The editorial concluded that British nutritional doctors, and undoubtedly those in America, knew so little about mineral nutrition that no one can begin to say which trace minerals are, or are not, important.

9.

ALCOHOL AND THE ADRENAL GLANDS

Dr. Abram Hoffer, the noted Canadian psychiatrist, in his introduction to my book, *Mental Health Through Nutrition*, said: "I have examined hundreds of patients and have found, as have many others, that every alcoholic tested had hypoglycemia. There was really no point in testing them any further, since there were no exceptions."

Dr. Tintera, who was a charter member of the New York Medical Committee on Alcoholism, and an authority on the endocrine treatment of alcholics, stated in one of his published medical papers: "Show me an alcoholic, any alcoholic, and I will show you adrenal glands exhausted by alcohol."

Most of us have grown accustomed to thinking of chronic alcoholics, who probably include six or seven million Americans, as suffering from a disease, *alcoholism*. We haven't given much thought to how alcoholism should or could be treated, and we have generally assumed that alcoholism must have been caused by some early emotional trauma and that it is the problem of the alcoholic and his psychiatrist, or of Alcoholics Anonymous, to get the alcoholic back on the right track.

The physicians who hold that alcoholism is not a disease in itself, but a symptom of the functional disturbance in the cortex of the adrenal glands, with the same mental abberations sometimes found in hypoglycemic states, have found that alcoholism responds well to the endocrine therapy.

Dr. Tintera, in a paper published in the *New York Journal of Medicine* on December 15, 1956, reported that he had successfully treated more than 200 alcoholics, many of whom had been members of Alcoholics Anonymous for several years. Dr. Tintera proceeded in those cases on the assumption that alcoholism, like hay fever, asthma, migraine, or hives, is a symptom of a glandular disorder. He does not discount the value of the wonderful work done by the Alcoholics Anonymous organization.

I have read every book I have been able to find relating to the work of Alcoholics Anonymous. Without going into detail as to how A.A. works or for what it stands, I know it has done more for mankind during the past 40 years than has any other similarly organized group in the history of the world during the same period of time.

Alcoholics call upon general practitioners to treat them for heart disease and cancer (in that order of frequency) more than for alcoholism. Doctors tell us, however, that alcoholism is growing and that unless the present trend is reversed, alcoholism will become one of the most common diseases with which the general practitioners or family doctors have to cope.

Now that we know more about alcoholism, the

social stigma has been partially removed from alchoholism, and some hospitals admit alcoholics as patients. Due to the crowded conditions prevailing in most hospitals, these patients are kept for only a limited time. I am told that in some of our larger cities hospital facilities for treating alcoholics as alcoholics, and not as merely physically ill persons, have been established. In many states however, there are no hospitals or adequate facilities available for the treatment of these people, particularly if they are without funds to pay for such care.

Throughout the country, we have many farms or "alcoholic sanitaria," privately run by lay management (usually alcoholics themselves), where the "patients," or whatever they are called, are mistreated and misguided; and then, when whatever funds the alcoholic or his family has are gone, he returns to to society worse off — if any change has occurred — than when he entered.

I think all physicians who have made an extensive study of alcoholism generally agree that the successful treatment of alcoholism requires the recognition that it has rightfully been placed in the classification of a psychosomatic disorder. However, physicians are not completely in agreement as to the part, if any, drug therapy, should and can play. This much can be said: those who contend that alcoholism is purely a psychic phenomenon are unable to show any appreciable percentage of recoveries through psychiatry alone. Those who contend that alcoholism is not primarily a psychic disorcer, but rather an organic disease referable to the men of internal medicine, are unable to show any better record of recoveries than are the psychiatrists.

Dr. Tintera said that endocrinology is a requisite for the consummate treatment of the disorder. He pointed out that it is a well-known fact that the last person to recognize an alcoholic problem is the alcoholic himself.

Without considering those patients brought, intoxicated, to the doctor by family pressure or a clash with the law, those who only desire to be sobered up, or those who come to the physician solely for help in getting over a hangover (without any intent of giving up drinking), Dr. Tintera went on to discuss those individuals who recognize they have an alcoholic problem and plead for help in getting over their craving for alcohol. He was talking about the patient who, after a long period of sobriety, wants to obtain permanent sobriety.

Dr. Tintera stated that the recovered alcoholic consults his doctor because he is dissatisfied with his way of life, even if he has maintained sobriety for years. His symptoms are an aggravation of those that initiated his drinking.

Even when they have remained "dry," as A.A. puts it, for years, alcoholics usually have insatiable desires for sweets or carbohydrates in some form. They are frequently introverted and anti-social; they are dependent individuals who must regain their confidence and a desire to be productive and useful. Unless the patient is willing to give up drinking completely, he is wasting his time and that of his doctor. Even if he believes he can limit his drinking to a weekend cocktail, the treatment will be a complete failure. Until such time as the patient has conceded that total and complete alcoholic restriction from then on is necessary, failure of treatment is inevitable.

The tests the doctor gives are more detailed than those discussed in prior chapters, since the physician must determine — either at the start of the treatment or later — the amount of liver damage, if any, caused by the prolonged drinking. He also carefully checks to see if there has been any damage to the patient's kidneys. Upon completion of a thorough physical examination and complete history, three laboratory tests are routinely given: (1) urinalysis, (2) complete blood count, and (3) a glucose tolerance test. If the patient is found to be suffering from hypoadrenocorticism, he is put on the anti hypoglycemia diet previously outlined, with one exception: it is a high protein, low carbohydrate, high fat diet, instead of the medium fat diet prescribed for non-alcoholic patients.

The patient is then given the adrenal cortex extract injections. As in other cases of hypoadrenocorticism, the length of the intervals between injections increases as the patient approaches the time when the injections may be discontinued.

Dr. Tintera believed that regular consultations of a psychiatric nature between the physician (generally a general practitioner or family doctor) and the patient, must continue indefinitely. The patient must be continually reassured by his doctor as he redirects him to a more fruitful outlook on life. There must be a rational medical explanation in layman's language of the emotional, psychological, hormonal ramifications of the patient's illness. When the patient is able to control and understand the hypoglycemic episodes discussed in prior chapters, he will be relieved of much of his tension.

It is a procedure that requires understanding and patience on the part of the physician, for he may expect some reverses as the treatment proceeds. Many times the patient, without returning to liquor, will indicate that he can't go through with the treatment; and there will be times when the patient is very depressed and needs more than usual reassurance. As the treatment progresses, the patient's entire outlook will improve; there will be lessening of his negativism and a reversal of the personality traits present at the beginning of the treatment.

Within the first few months of treatment, endocrine balance will be established. As the patient regains physiological, endocrinological, and mental balance, he becomes aware of his social obligations and loses his compulsions, apprehensions, and inhibitions. We then have a clear-thinking, calm, outgoing, and energetic individual.

The patient must be taught that if he allows his blood sugar to reach hypoglycemic levels again, many of his original emotional problems will return — along with a craving for carbohydrates, more specifically, alcohol.

Pyridoxine (vitamin B_6) is frequently given as a valuable adjunct in rehabilitating alcoholics. Although alcoholism has never been one of my problems, a dermatologist once prescribed vitamin B_6 supplement for a scaly, itching dermatitis which had been annoying me a long time. This vitamin supplement soon cured my skin condition. The only reason for mentioning this is that I have noticed that a number of alcoholics brought before me as a district judge on various charges had noticeable skin diseases on their faces, particularly around their eyes and ears.

Alcohol is the adrenals' number-one enemy. Someone born with strong adrenals will probably be able to drink heavily for a long time before he becomes an alcoholic. The chances are he can drink in moderation all of his life without alcohol injuring him seriously. If an individual was born with weak adrenals, or if his adrenals have been damaged by disease, he will not be able to drink very long until alcohol does him lasting damage.

We speculate why one man can drink heavily for years and not become an alcoholic, while another becomes an alcoholic after drinking a few years. To say that a person will become an alcoholic if he is a heavy drinker for a certain number of years is as absurd as to say a man will develop heart disease when his weight reaches a certain number of pounds over what is should be.

Body chemistry has no use for alcohol; its whole aim is to get rid of it. To do so, it must convert alcohol into carbon dioxide and water. This chemical conversion takes place largely in the liver and it continues as long as there is any alcohol in the body. The adrenal cores secrete their stress hormone; the whole system of endocrine glands is roused, and the adrenal casing hormones direct glucose into the blood from the liver, where the glucose has been stored as glycogen.

Blood sugar level goes up, so the islets of the pancreas pour insulin into the blood to lower it. One drink will keep this chemical chaos going for a few hours. If you drink no more than that you feel quite normal again after a brief letdown. The whiplashing the adrenals receive is not long and not severe, so the glands can recover quickly.

If you have a lot of drinks, you wind up with more or less exhausted adrenals and with what we call a hangover — a low blood sugar condition. You feel terrible, listless, tired and depressed, have a headache, and are unable to think clearly. If you don't drink again, your adrenals will recover in a day or a week (depending on the strength of your glands), and you will feel normal again.

But, for the man or woman who becomes an alcoholic, things don't work out that way. While the adrenals are still more or less exhusted, and while the blood sugar level is down, the individual starts drinking again in order to feel better; the same chemical process begins, and, unless he stops drinking, the person finally collapses. This is the chemical merry-go-round to which an alcoholic is chained.

As glycogen is taken from the liver without being replaced through proper nutrition, more fat collects in the liver. The alcoholic gets his calories from alcohol, and these calories are quickly metabolized. The inevitable result, unless drinking is at least temporarily stopped, is general physical collapse and probable death caused by a ruined liver and pancreas.

The physical basis of alcoholism is, then, a functional disturbance of the adrenals and a real, organic need for sugar. If that were all there is to alcoholism, it would be one of the easiest diseases of all to curb. All the doctor would need to do would be to put the alcoholic on a diet that places little strain on the adrenals and administer adrenal cortex extract until the adrenals rehabilitated themselves.

However, alcoholism is not that simple a disease. It involves the whole person, the body, the mind, and the emotions. After the alcoholic's physical craving for liquor is gone, treatment must continue until such time as the person's mental and emotional difficulties are under control. Dr. Tintera observed that an alcoholic, *any alcoholic,* can be sobered permanently if he has a strong enough will to stop drinking completely and forever. That doesn't mean he will have to continue with the adrenal cortex extract, but it does mean he may have to remain on the diet for an indefinite length of time.

I am sure you have known alcoholics who have stopped drinking and substituted sugar or sugar products for alcohol. The physical craving for alcohol will continue as long as the alcoholic keeps his chemical merry-go-round in motion, whether from alcohol or other quickly-absorbed carbohydrates, such as sugar, candies, pastries, sweetened soft drinks, cakes pies, cereals, potatoes, corn, dates, raisins, honey, and spaghetti. The adrenals and the islets of the pancreas will carry on their tug of war over lowering and raising the blood sugar level, and the alcoholic, although "dry," will feel miserable most of the time.

The view that alcoholism is a complicated disease, and not evidence of a depraved mind, is held by a minority — but certainly an enlightened minority — of our people. When we try to determine why any alcoholic started to drink, we have a difficult question to answer. When we ask why he continued to drink more and more as time went on, we have a more difficult question to answer. In trying to get the answers to some of these questions, I have talked with many alcoholics who have appeared in my courts.

Since my attitude toward these people has always been one of sympathy and not of condemnation, practically all of them have given me truthful answers, *as far as they knew,* even when I, as a trial judge, imposed penitentiary sentences for offenses they had committed. They could not explain their early problems, if any, because of my lack of psychiatric training and the lack of time for more than casual interviews.

I was astounded at the effects intoxication had on them. Alcohol, so they said, gave them a sense of importance, relieved their apprehensions and anxieties, and gave them a temporary feeling of well-being, a reversal of their usual feelings of inferiority. Some of them told me they thought they got drunk to punish themselves for something — they did not know what. I did not have to remind any of them that what they told me were rationalizations; they admitted that as a part of their answers. More than half of them said, in substance: "I know I am running from something; I don't know what it is." We can call these people cowards, but aren't we all cowards in some way or another?

Medical science is doing a wonderful work in helping alcoholics rehabilitate. I think some doctors' intitial approach is wrong. They tell an alcoholic that some day he will be able, or *perhaps* be able, to drink again. Their excuse for doing so is that they want to give the alcoholic something to "hang on to;" otherwise they fear he will never try to help himself.

I think a doctor should never lie to a patient unless it is necessary to save the patient's life or prevent immediate serious injury. If, in the back of his mind, the alcoholic believes he will be able to drink again, he is liable to cheat and believe he can fool his doctor by taking a drink or a few drinks without the doctor's knowledge.

Until an alcoholic knows that he has a drinking problem and will have it the rest of his life, and until he has absolutely and completely determined, without any reservation, to give up drinking forever, *he is beyond the help of medical science.* Doctors by the dozens have agreed with me on the statement I have just made. They have further agreed with me on these things:

1. The alcoholic must be made to understand that one drink any time and any place will again enslave him.

2. He must be told that every hour and every day he abstains he will more and more appreciate and enjoy the concrete benefits of a properly functioning glandular system; that people and the world will look better to him every day he goes without liquor. The temptation to take just a little drink is greatest at a time of stress or grief, and that is the most dangerous time. If the alcoholic gets by such a period without a drink, he wins a great victory.

3. There is no such a person as a "cured" or "recovered" alcoholic. The patient should be told that it will be impossible for him to always run from alcohol and that the best answer for him to give when would-be friends insist that he drink, is to tell them he is an alcoholic and can never drink again; then stick to it.

4. The physician should, in sympathetic and understandable language, explain to the patient the treatment and the reasons for the treatment.

5. Psychotherapy by the doctor is more important than medication and diet. While the physician must at all times have a sympathetic and understanding attitude, more help will come to the patient if he is the one who initiates the inquiries and attempts to answer his own questions. The alcoholic is

usually a sensitive person who resents any lecturing or sermonizing by his doctor or by members of his family.

6. Sometimes the husband or wife of an alcoholic needs counselling by the doctor; the spouse's attitude might have to be changed so that he or she will be able to assist in educating and directing the alcoholic to a new life of happiness, usefulness, and productivity.

Unless the physician likes people and has a sincere desire to help them, he will not be interested in trying to help an alcoholic rehabilitate himself. Every alcoholic who comes to a doctor with a sincere desire to be rehabilitated and a willingness to conform to whatever is required of him, presents a challenge to the doctor as great, if not greater, than the challenge which an unusual, delicate, and difficult operation presents to a great surgeon. If I had my life to live over, I would study medicine instead of law, so that I might be able to try to help do some of the things I have talked about in this chapter.

Doctors have observed that they never knew a diabetic who became an alcoholic. There are alcoholics, however, who have become diabetics. These people burdened their livers and pancreatic glands to such an extent that both became diseased, and the islands of Langerhans, that part of the pancreas that manufactures insulin, became unable to furnish normal daily amounts of insulin.

A well-known eastern physician wrote me: "I would not for a moment discount the wonderful work of Alcoholics Anonymous. They have dried up more men and women than have all of the doctors in America combined. However, every medical advisor to Alcoholics Anonymous I ever knew believed that the best way to rehabilitate alcoholics was by the glandular treatment and psychotherapy."

The cost to the nation caused by the excessive use of alcohol is now estimated to be more than a billion dollars annually. This is only a part of the overall cost. The thousands upon thousands of divorce cases that have gone through my courts have provided me with first-hand information about the tragedies, the suffering, and the ruined lives of those who never drank but were the victims of alcoholism as much as, if not more than, the alcoholics themselves.

There is no escaping the responsibility we all have for the high rate of alcoholism in this nation. We must recognize the social anomaly that makes social drinking respectable and leads a weak and dependent character into alcoholism. We salve our consciences by saying, "it's a free country," the one who will later become an alcoholic, "doesn't have to drink unless he wants to do so," and, after all, "it's really none of our business who drinks or how much he drinks."

After we have furnished the opportunity and encouraged a weak and dependent individual to become an alcoholic, we become rather high and mighty in our attitude toward him. "He's gotten himself in that condition; let him get out of it." It's not difficult for us to become self-righteous about our social drinking. Sometimes we become bighearted in our willingness to help our former drinking friends. If they don't have any money to get help for themselves, which we know is often the case, we don't grumble too much about paying our share of taxes for public institutions to help the destitute alcoholics. I am sure that our hypocrisy about our responsibility for some of the results of social drinking is at least partially responsible for the callous manner in which we treat most alcoholics.

Doctors tell us alcohol is not addicting, like morphine and cocaine, but it is definitely habit-forming. It is dangerous because it is connected with a ritual, such as communal drinking, which has social approbation. Why then does the alcoholic apparently have such an uncontrollable appetite for liquor? If the forces of psychological stimulation are the sole causes of irresistible craving for alcohol, how can we explain the hangover or the alcoholic's inability to keep from pouring liquor into his body when he knows that no pleasure, only suffering, can come to him?

Never having drunk much liquor, I can only base my conclusions on my own experiences. Similarly, under the established rules of evidence, a lay witness may state opinions in courts of law if he first states the facts upon which his opinions are based. Many, many times I have had as uncontrollable a desire for sugar as any alcoholic ever had for liquor. The more sugar I ate, the more sugar I wanted. Because I was sober, I knew better than the alcoholic what sugar would do to me.

No advocate of the theory that alcoholism is psychic and psychic only will ever be able to convince me that my uncontrollable craving for sugar was all psychological. My body was crying out for food; although I was overweight, I was at least partially starving. When I ate sugar, the glucose that entered my bloodstream made me feel good.

Fortunately for me, I went for the sugar instead of the alcohol. I believe that I had as many emotional and mental problems to face when I reached maturity as does the average person who becomes an alcoholic. Yet, my problems were easier to solve than they would have been had I become an alcoholic, because sugar or other ordinary carbohydrate food does not damage the body, the brain, the mind, and the personality as alcohol does.

When I went on the antihypoglycemic diet and began taking the adrenal cortex injections, my problem was simple — regaining my health. Sugar had done no damage to me that could not be repaired easily and in a fairly short time.

At the beginning of any rehabilitation program, the alcoholic's problems are complex and difficult. His body chemistry was out of order to begin with, and by drinking he brought upon himself all the ills of alcoholism. He has a rough road ahead of him, even if every person he meets is kind, considerate, and sympathetic. Most of us are moralists when dealing with the other person's faults and weaknesses. We are far more charitable with our own faults and weaknesses than we are with those of our friends and relatives. The alcoholic frequently finds himself a world apart, where few are tolerant, sympathetic, or kind to him.

After he no longer has a physical need for liquor and has determined, with all the will power he possesses, never to take another drink, the alcoholic is, in some ways, like a little child learning to walk. He falters, he stumbles, he may even fall down; but every day he is more determined than ever to succeed in conquering his alcoholism. The most despicable character I can think of is one who deliberately does something to impede the alcoholic in his determination to "walk as he once did."

To my way of thinking, the secret of the success of Alcoholics Anonymous is its humanness; it gives the new member the feeling — perhaps for the first time in years — that he has friends who understand and appreciate what he is up against. It is a form of mass psychotherapy conducted by laymen who, by nature, are sympathetic to their fellow men.

A.A. was not organized to furnish medical treatment to its members; that they must get themselves. However, it has given the members of America's low and middle income classes the opportunity, that formerly only the rich could afford, to rebuild their lives. A.A. is a great success if for no other reason than that it is effective among the alcoholics who seek its aid.

10.

TRACKING DOWN THE
NUMBER ONE KILLER

Every physician who has successfully treated allergy cases with the antihypoglycemia diet and adrenal cortex extract injections has observed the improvement in the general health of his patients.

Doctors with whom I have corresponded have commented on how the antihypoglycemia diet reduced the amount of cholesterol in the bloodstream. Physicians have been telling us for years that lowering cholesterol prevents and sometimes cures atherosclerosis, a condition where blood passages are narrowed, with the result that clots adhere to the linings of the vessels, stopping the normal flow of blood to the heart. This causes what the doctors refer to as a "coronary occlusion," a "myocardial infarction," or what the layman speaks of as a "heart attack."

When I began my research, I was only interested in allergy cases; however, when both patients and doctors told me, in substance, that the diet and medication discussed in prior chapters seemed to prevent and hasten recovery from coronary attacks, I was intrigued. Because so many judges and lawyers have recently suffered heart attacks, I was anxious to know why a low carbohydrate and high protein diet might be beneficial in preventing attacks of the nation's "number one killer." coronary heart disease.

The answers given me by both doctors and laymen were convincing. They suggested that the clearing of fat and other sludge from the bloodstream was promoted by one or more of the following factors: (1) Eliminating pies, cakes, and other pastries from the diet, thus reducing the fat intake. (2) A diet rich in fruits and vegetables with a high vitamin C content, which, along with increased amounts of other vitamins, may be beneficial. (3) Attaining and maintaining normal weight while on the diet. (4) Reducing tensions and anxieties by means of diet and medication. (The effect is much the same as that of tranquilizing drugs — but without unfavorable side effects.)

A team of physicians in California, including Dr. Meyer Friedman and Dr. Ray H. Rosenman, both cardiologists, and Dr. Sanford O. Byers, a biochemist, have worked for years to determine the causes of coronary heart disease. These physicians had thousands of business executives as volunteers and made what was probably the most complete, massive study undertaken in the medical battle against coronary attacks.

Late in 1964, the *Journal of the American Medical Association* reported the findings of this medical team. These physicians discovered that the administration of ACTH (adrenocorticotropin) to their volunteers after rich meals quickly cleared fat from the bloodstream. Tests made on these volunteers after they had been given the same rich food but not the ACTH showed that some of the fat remained in the bloodstream as long as 24 hours after the meals had been eaten.

Tests made by these California specialists on persons whose adrenal glands had been removed showed conclusively that ACTH by itself did not clear the bloodstream after rich meals.

As was observed in a prior chapter, ACTH stimulates the adrenals to produce more hormones. From the report of Drs. Friedman, Rosenman and Byers, we know that *malfunction of the adrenal glands is one of the causes of coronary heart disease.* These California doctors and many others are attempting to identify the adrenal hormone that apparently clears the bloodstream of excess fats and cholesterol. When this hormone is discovered, it will, without doubt, be produced synthetically and made available to physicians. Further testing will be necessary to determine whether the synthetic hormone can safely be used in coronary heart disease cases.

When Drs. Friedman and Rosenman made a report in 1958 to the American Heart Association that their tests had indicated that blood cholesterol level was not controlled solely by diet, they were greeted with dead silence.

It is axiomatic that if the adrenals are manufacturing all of their hormones in sufficient quantities, there is no necessity for stimulating them with ACTH.

How far medical researchers will go in proving that adequate hormone production by the adrenal glands prevents and, when induced, can cure a myriad of diseases, is as much the guess of one person as it is of another. It would appear that even now, with the medical knowledge of hypoglycemia and hypoadrenocorticism available to physicians, heart disease need not continue to be the nation's number one killer.

It seems to me that if we had a few large hypoglycemia foundations in America, it would not take long for physicians to be able to tell us the role, if any, that our adrenals play in our illnesses. Even before the eminent California doctors made their momentous discovery that some unknown hormone from the adrenal glands is responsible for removing fat, calcium, and other sludge from our bloodstreams, other physicians, sometimes family doctors, had become convinced that the adrenals had something to do with preventing and curing heart disease. These doctors did not have the time, the money, or the facilities to make the massive tests of the California physicians.

I have not attempted to summarize all of the findings and conclusions of Dr. Friedman and Dr. Rosenman. They found that aggressive, hard-driving men are subject to heart attack, and also that among men prone to coronary disease, high fat levels build up in the bloodstream. They have demonstrated that heart attacks can be fairly accurately predicted in men who showed no clinical evidence of coronary disease. Their report, in part, read: "The frequent heart attack after a heavy meal now becomes explicable to us."

I do not contend that the low carbohydrate, high protein diet and adrenal cortex extract medication constitute a "cure-all" for all diseases, but I am hopeful that in the next several years much medical research will be done to determine the role of the adrenal glands in all kinds of disease. I believe that if and when this is done, some of the reports will be as startling to both physicians and laymen as were the published results of the tests made by Dr. Friedman and Dr. Rosenman.

We are told that close to 25 million people in the nation are hypertensive, or have high blood pressure. The insurance companies estimate that 40 million hypertensives may be a more accurate estimate.

The first number of a blood-pressure reading is the systolic — the measurement in millimeters of mercury of the force of the column of blood as it leaves the heart and strikes the walls of the first big blood vessel, the aorta. The bottom number is the diastolic reading — the measurement in millimeters of mercury of the resistance this column of blood must overcome to pass through the smaller blood vessels. So we say the systolic pressure is a measure of force and the diastolic pressure is a measure of resistance.

Until late in the sixties physicians were taught that a normal, systolic reading should be 100 added to our age, and the diastolic reading was much more important than a systolic reading.

As a result of a 20-year study by the United States Public Health Service on a whole town, commonly called the "Framingham Study," and released a few years back, doctors are now taught the upper reading (systolic) should not exceed 140, and lower reading (diastolic) should never be more than 90, and that systolic pressure is as important as diastolic.

Your blood pressure can vary from hour to hour— go up or down, depending on exertion, emotional and other factors. Only by repeated readings under relaxed conditions can a doctor correctly diagnose blood pressure. That is why you should not be alarmed about hypertension solely as the result of a free blood-pressure test made in a supermarket, or on the street. Your doctor may make many tests before he can decide whether you are, or are not, hypertensive.

The only part of your body where a physician can actually see the blood vessels is by looking at the back of the eye through an ophthalmoscope. When you had your last eye examination for possible change of glasses, your ophthamologist may have told you that you had hardening of the arteries, broken blood vessels or other symptoms of high blood pressure.

Some people with high blood pressure feel fine and have no symptoms. Others complain of headaches, dizziness, fatigue or shortness of breath, without knowing they are hypertensive. Insurance company physicians tell us that from 35 to 50 per cent of all hypertensives are unaware of their high blood pressure.

Except for cardiologists and obstetricians, physicians have been negligent about checking the blood pressure of patients. Hypertensives do not have their blood pressure checked as often as it should be checked.

Hypertension is usually a major contributing factor to coronary-artery disease. Since *most abnormal blood sugar sufferers die from some form of cardiovascular disease, it is imperative that we avoid, if at all possible, those things that bring on stroke, heart failure and other coronary-artery diseases.*

Low blood pressure is consistent with longevity, but accidents, serious illness, sudden emotional problems and some unknown factors can cause one with low blood pressure to become hypertensive.

Once you are hypertensive, you should have the services of a physician. Your doctor will prescribe drugs, insist that you reduce if you are overweight, and probably recommend a low-salt diet. Fortunately, hypertension is easy to diagnose and not difficult to treat.

What can we do so our friends will not say: "He was so young and his death so unnecessary?" We know that we cannot follow all of the recommendations of the cardiologists because they do not agree as to the causes of coronary death. For example, we are told that polyunsaturated fats will protect us from premature heart attack. Yet the classic, long-term "Framingham Study" reported: ". . .there is no discernible association between reported diet intake and serum cholesterol level."

We all know the usual rules given to avoid heart attacks and strokes:

1. Eat polyunsaturated fats.
2. Avoid stress, tension and anxiety.
3. Take off weight, if too heavy.
4. Stop smoking cigarettes.
5. Keep blood pressure within normal limits.
6. Get some exercise each day.
7. Don't drink alcoholic beverages to excess.
8. Get sufficient sleep.

Some foods are better than others for cardiovascular health. The antihypoglycemia diet of Chapter 3 is excellent to follow to avoid coronary disease. Nutritionists, lay and medical, believe the diet should be supplemented with vitamins and minerals.

There are some foods I want to especially recommend that you eat to keep your heart and blood vessels young and healthy. These are:

Apples. Our grandparents knew that "an apple a day keeps the doctor away." We know now that it is the pectin in apples and some other fruits that makes them so valuable as a health food. Dr. Ancel Keys, nutritional expert, cited experiments made in 1960 to show that pectin lowers blood cholesterol. (See *Proceedings of the Society for Experimental Biology and Medicine,* 1961).

Grant Palmer and David Dixon reported in the June, 1966, *American Journal of Clinical Nutrition* that men with normal cholesterol levels, when pectin was added to their diet, had lower cholesterol levels.

The Lancet, April 15, 1975, reported on a study funded by the British Heart Association, and still underway, showing that pectin lowers cholesterol levels.

Physicians do not know how pectin lowers cholesterol in the blood. The soundest theory advanced is that it stops the intestine from absorbing fatty acids so they pass out of the body without entering the bloodstream.

Dr. Ancel Keys summed it all up in this sentence: "It appears probable, however, that the high consumption of fruits, including apples, by some populations, helps to explain the low cholesterol values of those populations."

There are so many ways to eat apples that one should never get tired of them. Eat them raw or cooked, as a salad food, as a part of the main meal or as a dessert. Apple juice can be taken any time. Italian researchers found that apple sauce stabilized cholesterol levels. Apple pectin tablets are available and inexpensive. If you eat raw apples, I suggest you peel them to get rid of the poisons from spraying.

Beans. In their book, *The Benevolent Bean*, Margaret and Ancel Keys made a study of the relationship of the low coronary rate in Italy and the Italians' love of beans. Dr. Ancel Keys experimented with Minnesota men who ate, as Dr. Keys reported, "the leafy vegetables, the abundant fruits, the beans and other leguminous seeds so prominent in the daily diet of Naples." As a result, the cholesterol level of the Minnesota men fell from an average of 225 to 165, which is the cholesterol level of the average Neapolitan. "If you happen to be interested in cholesterol control, beans or any leguminous seeds merit a prominent place in your diet," said Dr. Keys.

Asparagus. Aspartic acid is one of the nonessential amino acids. Two French physicians, Drs. M. Lamarche and R. Royer, after animal experimentation, found that aspartic acid slows down the heart in a distress situation. What these doctors did was to partially cut off the supply of oxygen to the heart, causing it to beat faster, and then introduce aspartic acid in the bloodstream. This caused a slowing down of beats per minute.

Other European doctors found that aspartic acid decreases fatigue and increases available energy. They have recommended that further studies be made to treat human coronary insufficiency with aspartic acid since it is known to be an important detoxifier. Your heart will love asparagus!

Lecithin. This important food has been found useful in fighting cholesterol. It is found in natural vegetable oils, beef liver, brains, kidneys, beef heart, egg yolk, wheat germ, nuts and seeds. Soybeans are an excellent source of lecithin.

Researchers have shown that lecithin breaks down cholesterol into small particles that move easily in the bloodstream with no harm resulting. Fats, when hydrogenated, lose lecithin, so cholesterol in hydrogenated fats is dangerous because it does not have protective lecithin. The cholesterol from fats without lecithin collects on the arterial walls and heart disease follows.

An article in the January, 1958, *Geriatrics* reported that two tablespoons of lecithin given daily to patients with high cholesterol and high blood pressure reduced the cholesterol level 41 per cent in 13 out of 15 patients.

Dr. Lester M. Morrison, prominent Los Angeles physician, recently said: "There seems to be good evidence now in very high concentrations lecithin can dissolve the fatty plaques in the arteries."

Drs. Pottenger and Krohn, in the *American Journal of Digestive Diseases*, (April, 1962) told how they put their patients with high blood pressure on diets high in cholesterol and lecithin made from soybeans. "The blood cholesterol showed a marked decrease in 79 per cent of the patients who took the lecithin," the report said.

Many more recent medical articles attest the effectiveness of lecithin to reduce cholesterol levels and prevent the accumulation of hard gallstones.

For those who don't want extra calories, cheap lecithin capsules, which are quite effective, are available.

We hear much about low-salt diets to reduce blood pressure. In some unknown way, a duel seems to be fought in the body between sodium (salt) and potassium. When salt seems to win, the supply of potassium in the body is low; when potassium predominates, the amount of salt is reduced.

Dr. Samuel Bellet in his book, *Potassium; Cardiac Aspects, the Role of Potassium in Health and Disease*, reported that animals on diets low in potassium, after several weeks, showed evidence of myocardial necrosis of the heart. He said that a heart lesion in animals can be produced in four days with a diet high in salt and low in potassium.

Dr. W.A. Krehl said in *Nutrition in Clinical Medicine*, (June 22, 1966): "If food habits had always been sound, the event of potassium deficiency and depletion would not have developed as a major medical problem."

Drs. J. Yerushalmy and Herman Hilleboe, in the June 15, 1957, *New York State Journal of Medicine* presented evidence that in countries where fat consumption is the same as ours, but where people eat a richer potassium diet than in the United States, the mortality rate for heart disease is slightly over one third of that in this nation.

Foods high in potassium are tomato catsup, brewer's yeast, wheat germ, soybeans, bran, dry nonfat milk, nuts and spinach.

Doctors do not recommend a low salt diet for patients with low blood pressure, and pregnant women.

The August 14, 1974, *Journal of the American Medical Association* quoted with approval from an article by Dr. D.P. Burkitt and associates, as follows: "Evidence is accumulating that shows the removal of fiber (such as the bran removed from the white flour) from the diet, raises serum cholesterol levels, a process that predisposes to coronary heart disease."

Physicians who for years have advocated a bland, highly refined food diet are taking a "second look" at the foods our ancestors ate when cerebral thrombosis, myocardial infarction and other cardiovascular diseases were unknown to doctors.

I am sure many of you will remember when Dr. Paul Dudley White, who was President Eisenhower's physician following his heart attack, said: "When I graduated from medical school in 1911, I had never heard of coronary thrombosis, which is one of the chief threats to life in the United States today — an astounding development in one's own lifetime! There can be no doubt but that coronary heart disease has reached epidemic proportions in the United States, where it is now responsible for more than 50 per cent of all deaths. . . The truth is, an ever-increasing number of young men are being struck down before the age of 40 (including a large number of physicians), at the time they are most needed by their families and when they are prepared to make their greatest contribution to society."

11.

YOU MAY BECOME A DIABETIC

Dr. Charles Weller, well-known diabetes specialist, said in his book, *The New Way to Live With Diabetes:* "Hypoglycemia frequently precedes diabetes." He went on to say: "...patients maintain their hypoglycemia for a time, but diabetes...then sets in."

Other medical writers have commented on the relationship between hypoglycemia and diabetes and that a considerable per cent of hypoglycemics become diabetics.

The symptoms of diabetes first noticed usually are:

1. Increased thirst and appetite.

2. Frequent urination.

3. A dry mouth, which is also present in hypoglycemia cases.

Other symptoms are:

(a) Changes in vision.

(b) Weight loss.

(c) Frequent fatigue.

(d) Cuts and bruises which heal slowly.

(e) Drowsiness.

(f) Pains or cramps in the fingers and toes.

(g) Sugar in the urine.

(h) Itching of the skin.

Practically all hypoglycemics who become diabetics are known as *adult* or *maturity-onset* diabetics. This type of diabetes is usually discovered in some casual way, as an examination for an insurance policy, a testing for eye glasses or a routine physical checkup.

Fortunately, diabetes developed by adults usually is not severe and can be controlled without insulin by a *strict adherence to diet* and keeping the weight down.

Unfortunately, the diagnosis of adult diabetes is not as easy as that of juvenile diabetes. A physician will ordinarily use a blood sugar or glucose tolerance test, or a series of such tests, to confirm diabetes.

The maturity-onset diabetic may not have a lack of insulin, but something in his body impedes the insulin activity he needs for proper carbohydrate metabolism.

Some overweight diabetics do not have enough insulin production to take care of their carbohydrates. In such cases a return to normal weight will correct the diabetic symptoms and all such a diabetic has to do is to keep his weight down by restricting the carbohydrate intake.

There is now no known cure for diabetes — it is for life — but a person who becomes diabetic as an adult should be able to function as well and live as long and fully as a non-diabetic, provided he keeps his weight normal, or slightly below normal, is careful of his diet and takes a reasonable amount of exercise. Severe stress, as with the loss of a job, a serious accident, a family breakup or a serious infection, may worsen his condition to where he may have to temporarily have medication.

Some overweight diabetics' blood sugar will remain

lower without insulin, and insulin causes them to gain weight. As Dr. Weller said in the book referred to earlier, "The key to successful treatment of overweight diabetics is that insulin should not be used, lest the patient's weight increase and thus worsen the disease."

What I am saying is that excess weight causes an increased demand for insulin, and the more fat one has the more insulin his body requires. Insulin is the most fat-producing hormone known. The vicious cycle needs to be broken if the blood sugar of the adult who developed diabetes is to be normal.

Dr. T.S. Danowski, a distinguished authority on diabetes, in his book, *Diabetes as a Way of Life*, said: "...virtually 100 per cent of the definitely overweight adult patients whose body weight is reduced to normal can be treated completely by dietary restriction without insulin. The same desirable effects can be achieved in some adults with mild diabetes who are not overweight."

Dr. Henry Dolger, another great diabetic specialist, in *How to Live With Diabetes*, told us that with non-obese adult diabetics with mild diabetes, "...the simple omission of concentrated sugars, pastry, and soft drinks is often enough. This is especially true of elderly individuals."

Dr. Dolger said that many mild diabetics "...need not bother with complicated diets at all. They can be treated by omitting from their meals sugars, syrups, pastry and soft drinks..."

All medical nutritionists agree that everyone, regardless of his blood sugar condition, should have a minimum of 100 grams of carbohydrates daily. They also agree that diabetics and hypoglycemics should eat those carbohydrates which are slowly absorbed in the bloodstream.

What about fats? The underweight "hypoglycemia-turned" diabetic need not worry about eating a reasonable amount of fats while shunning most of the carbohydrates. The overweight middle-aged housewife must drastically cut down on both fats and carbohydrates until she has her weight at the proper level.

While a diabetic need not be a food chemist, all authorities agree that the diabetic should know as much about his disease, nutrition and medication (if and when needed) as his physician. This doesn't mean he should be his own doctor, as he should be regularly examined and tested by his physician. The diabetic who is so ignorant of all these things — nutrition, the various kinds of diabetes, the problems of diabetics, the complications of diabetes, the tests for management of diabetes, when a diabetic should have insulin or an oral drug to control diabetes, what makes diabetes worse and dozens of other questions that will come to him, is in for a lot of trouble if he expects to find a doctor in this day and age who has time to answer all of his questions.

Every person in the nation faces blood vessel hazards. The one with diabetes may be subject to these additional hazards:

1. Special changes may occur in the blood vessels of the eyes, the kidneys and other body organs.

2. Cardiovascular diseases usually associated with age may appear earlier and be more extensive.

3. The protection from heart attacks by being a female may be lost.

This does not mean any of these things *will happen.*

It does mean the diabetic who wants to lead a long and worthwhile life has no choice except to keep his diabetes under control. It means a knowledge of the values of minerals, vitamins and exercise to all — those with low, high or normal blood sugar.

The cause of diabetes is still apparently unknown, but physicians were taught these things in medical schools:

1. Anyone can get diabetes, but adults are more likely than children to have it.

2. These persons are more likely than others to become diabetics:

(a) One from a diabetic family.

(b) An overweight individual.

(c) A woman rather than a man.

Hypoglycemia has been wrongfully diagnosed as diabetes, and I am certain that some hypoglycemics have been killed with insulin. The antihypoglycemia diet is nearly the same as the diet for diabetes (except the latter stresses weight reduction).

As Dr. Weller said in his book heretofore referred to, "diabetic foods" found in supermarkets are misleading as most of them contain sugar. Unless the label states that the food has no sugar, it is "off limits" to the diabetic.

The future of the "hypoglycemia-turned" diabetic becomes brighter each year. In 1974 researchers reported that a deficiency in the diet of a trace mineral, chromium, causes (a) elevated cholesterol blood levels, and (b) inability to handle glucose efficiently — a mild form of diabetes. Nations with high chromium in the diet have less heart attacks and a lower incidence of adult diabetes than do those with lower chromium levels.

Dr. Richard J. Doisy and associates reported in *Modern Medicine*, (September 16, 1974) that brewer's yeast, a rich source of chromium, fed to young people, some diabetics, decreased the need for insulin to keep blood sugar within bounds. Other researchers have noted that to be effective with mild diabetes, more brewer's yeast must be taken with meals than is recommended for vitamin deficiency.

If you are an adult diabetic, I suggest you try brewer's yeast, a harmless and cheap food that can be bought in powder or tablet form. As Dr. Doisy pointed out, individuals have different metabolic requirements, so an adult may need up to 20 grams, or two and a half tablespoonfuls daily of brewer's yeast.

I certainly don't recommend diabetes as a cure for allergies, but, as might be expected, diabetics do not suffer from allergies to the same extent as do hypoglycemics.

12.

A TREATMENT THAT CURES ALLERGIES

We who have gotten over our allergies by a treatment so new that more than half of our practicing physicians readily admit they know little or nothing about it, owe a tremendous debt of gratitude to the medical pioneers in hypoglycemia and hypoadrenocorticism. They have not received the recognition they so justly deserve from the public or from the medical associations.

A letter from a professor at Massachusetts Institute of Technology is indicative of what is being done in all parts of the nation by physicians who have the courage, the knowledge, and the determination to restore health to our long-suffering hypoadrenocortics. The letter reads:

June 13, 1963

Dear Judge Blaine:

I am pleased to respond to your letter.

My eldest daughter Martha was essentially bedridden, had no appetite, suffered from insomnia, and was seriously underdeveloped for her age, which was then eight years. Her condition derived from chronic asthma, which had

144

plagued her from approximately her first birthday and which had made impossible any of the physical activity normal for a young child; indeed, she missed over half of the first three years of school because of colds, flu, respiratory infections, and general sickliness. During this period, we continually consulted with the best allergy specialists available in Boston, submitting her to innumerable tests, treatments, and medications, all of which became progressively less effective. Compounding our difficulty was the fact that another child in our family of five daughters was exhibiting similar though less severe symptoms, as was my wife also; in many respects our home resembled a dispensary, with at least one, and usually several, persons ill and taking medicine against respiratory infection.

Using results of tests performed here at the Children's Medical Center and his supplementary personal observations, a physician diagnosed Martha's condition as extreme hypoadrenocorticism, thoroughly investigated our respective families' histories as related to and confirming her trouble, and commenced treatment of the child. Melodramatic though it may sound, the effects were immediately obvious. On the four-hour trip by auto to this doctor's office, she lay on an improvised bunk on the rear seat of the car with very little energy, appetite, or interest, and I carried her bodily, over my shoulder, from the parking lot into his office. Perhaps six hours later, when we were halfway home, she complained of hunger, walked unaided from the car to a roadside restaurant, ate a plateful of fried hamburgers and drank several glasses of milk, returned to the car unaided, and promptly fell asleep for the remainder of the journey.

Over the next several years, under this doctor's continued care and with the assistance of our local physician, Martha has continued to prosper; today she is robust, very athletic, rarely ill from any cause, does very well in her schoolwork, has an almost voracious appetite and could accurately be described as cured of asthma. The same can be said of her younger sister and of my wife; our entire family, by following the prescribed diet, now enjoys an unusually steady state of good health; and if any child needs to remain home from school for a day, or requires bed rest, it is something of an event — so much so that all of their teachers, with no prompting, have individually commented upon the unusual attendance records of all the children. To say we never become sick would be an exaggeration, but compared to our previous situation, the present one is a radical transformation for the better.

Perhaps because of my education and professional activities, I consistently evaluate a theory or an action by the results it produces and the effect it creates. The conventional treatments were not effective with my family; the care given produced the desired results in the three instances known to me intimately. Thus, I conclude that the analysis of the malfunction and treatment of it are correct. . .

Another letter came to me from a student with both a bachelor's degree and a master's degree, and who is now working toward his doctorate at Columbia University. The letter follows:

July 8, 1963

Dear Judge Blaine:

I have had an asthmatic condition all of my twenty-five years, having inherited same from my father. I can vividly recall how continually I suffered in my boyhood and adolescent days in Tennessee — not just for hours or a few days, but sometimes for as many as two consecutive weeks, particularly in the summer. Asthma powder and muscular injections of adrenalin provided my only

intermittent relief. Otherwise, I was practically immo-
bilized.

Somehow, I thought that all of this would end when I
moved to Buffalo, New York, in 1951, at the age of 14.
But it did not. I continued to have persistent wheezing
and shortness of breath, along with severe attacks from
time to time.

On occasion of one of the latter in 1955, I met an
allergist; and this time, I not only thought that it all
would end; I just knew that it would. Thus allergy tests
and subsequent immunization treatments were begun in
optimism, but the optimism proved to be only partially
warranted. Yes, I was helped. The severe attacks became
scattered to the point of having only about one a year for
the last few years (1960-62). Only, the wheezing and
shortness of breath continued as before, the difference
being that I was able to control them better. But so
doing required the continual use of a nebulizer and antihistamines. In fact, I do not recall a single day on which
I did not use my nebulizer!

This was my state of health when I came to school in
New York City in September, 1962. And unlike when I
left Tennessee, I had no hope of a change this time; but,
as fate would have it, change came anyway.

A physician began treating me in October, and change
began immediately. On the very next day after I received
my first treatment, I did not, for the first time since 1955,
use my nebulizer or take an antihistamine. Also, within
that first week, my shortness of breath became less pro-
nounced. Even more, within a two-week period, I began
to notice that I could read without getting as tired, that
I could type without making as many errors, and that I
could relax while writing. My condition, incidentally,
had become such that my hand muscles would tighten
when I wrote, or my hands would become very unsteady.

Today, ten months later, these changes persist. Wheezing and shortness of breath are things that I don't even think about any more. I work long hours (doing mental work) without becoming abnormally tired; I write without being nervous; and I type with greater accuracy and confidence. Additionally, my once pointed chest is beginning to flatten and broaden, and I'm gradually doing what I once thought was impossible for me, namely, gaining weight. Hence, for the first time in my life, I know what it is like to feel normal, to feel well, as it were.

Watching these changes unfold has been a source of great joy. Seeing, feeling, and yes, knowing that I am being transformed into a new being have given me a different image; vis-a-vis my fellow man, I no longer feel a hopeless sense of inadequacy.

Admittedly, I thought that I just couldn't live on the diet. How, I pondered, can I do without ice cream, pie, and all of the rest? But now, just as with wheezing and shortness of breath, I don't even think about it any more. In fact, I like it; the sacrifice involved gives me a sense of elevation.

You, therefore, can see that my own case history does help to justify the need for the popularity of your prospective book. To limit this discovery to the benefit of a few would be an inexcusable loss to the human race. Accordingly, I again congratulate you for undertaking your task, and wish you supreme success.

In all, Dr. Gyland treated over 1,000 cases in his seven years. He addressed the American Medical Association in New York City in 1957, and the Southern Medical Society in New Orleans in 1958. At the latter meeting, he showed the effect of functional hypoglycemia on skin, showing colored slides of skin conditions, before and after treatment. When the whole person was treated, the neurodermatitis got well.

Dr. Gyland's cholesterol on August 29, 1952, was 476. This was considered dangerously high at the clinic. They recommended a high protein, low fat diet. However, Dr. Gyland found the high fat diet keeps the pancreas from overactivity, and he felt that this was the more dangerous condition. So he continued to eat his two eggs for breakfast and to have a high protein, moderate fat diet, mostly vegetable fat. He was on no medicine to lower his cholesterol, but on October 7, 1953, it had dropped to 350, and on May 15, 1954, it was 250, and on September 22, 1955, it was 208. This was another indication that his body was functioning normally. He adhered strictly to the Seale Harris diet, plus his modification of it, and did not even take decaffeinated coffee or weak tea. Medicines often contain caffeine and their use is forbidden. He found the injections of . . . [trade name of calcium omitted] to be very beneficial. He also found that patients must be off tranquilizers for five days prior to the six-hour glucose tolerance test, since the use of tranquilizers gave a patient an abnormally high curve, a curve quite different from the curve made from the test on the patient when tranquilizers were discontinued.

His final illness followed an operation on his aorta. My present work is in the field of nutrition among the elderly, and it is challenging, too.

Sincerely,

RUTH GYLAND

Quite accidentally, I came across a paper published in July, 1935, in *California and Western Medicine*, reporting a talk made early that year before the General Medicine Section of the California Medical Association. The subject of the paper was: "The Treatment of Asthma, with Special Reference to the Oral Use of the Adrenal Hormones and Sodium Chloride."

A letter of inquiry disclosed that the author was still living and a distinguished and active member of the California medical profession.

The remarkable thing about this paper is that it is about 15 years ahead of most other articles I have been able to find relating to the use of adrenal hormones in the treatment of allergies. I secured permission from this physician to use any or all of his 1935 article in this book. I quote from the paper:

> In August, 1932, we began feeding whole beef adrenal glands to a group of patients . . . These were administered within a few hours from the time they were removed from the animals. Our reason for this was because of the various reports connecting this condition with adrenal deficiency. The improvement in their energy and sense of well-being was very definite. In September, 1932, a child whom we were treating had been suffering from continuous asthma for several months and was completely exhausted. With the idea that we might at least relieve his exhaustion, we gave him seven grams of whole raw beef adrenal gland, which was first ground and mixed with peanut butter. That night the child became free from asthma and remained so for three days. This gave the impetus to the studies leading up to the present report. Later, we began extracting the cortical hormone . . .

Several medical articles referred to the experiences of the late Dr. Stephen Gyland of Tampa, Florida. I wrote Dr. Gyland's widow and asked her to give me a letter with permission to use it in this publication. Her letter is as follows:

Dear Judge Blaine:

I am writing you concerning the illness and spectacular recovery of Stephen Gyland, M.D., my late husband.

In 1949, he began to have blackout spells which doctors he consulted could not account for. He had had severe tachycardia (racing heart) for several years previous to this, and went through two large northern clinics, where no reason could be found except "overwork." He was advised to give up his more taxing medical work and drink liquor to relieve the tachycardia. He did both with no help; but of course, the drinks could cause harm.

Another complaint was severe headaches, from which he had suffered for 20 years. These were diagnosed as "tension headaches," with no prescription except less work. His fatigue was great, and he woke up in the mornings more tired than when he went to bed. He was a kind, conscientious, understanding Christian general practitioner, so [he] was in great demand.

About '49 he also developed such severe arthritis in his legs and hands that he had to give up golf. Blurred and double vision plagued him and he became depressed — a complete change of personality.

He was given tests for suspected brain tumor. A 2-hour glucose tolerance test showed that his blood sugar rose to almost 280. Both he and his doctor decided that small doses of insulin might help, and they did temporarily, but he soon became almost incapacitated again. He shook like a leaf and staggered when he walked.

In 1952 our son was interning at a fine medical school center and insisted that his dad should come there for more tests, which Dr. Gyland, Sr. underwent for eleven days.

At the conclusion, the neuroligist said to him, "You

are finished for life. You will never see another patient. You have cerebral arteriosclerosis." The medical doctor who coordinated all the work done was more gentle and said, "Come back in six months and let us see you then. You don't have diabetes, so quit taking insulin. Your future is in the hands of the Lord."

This doctor had ordered a six-hour glucose tolerance test which showed a rise to 265 and a rapid drop to 76. He said it was the "craziest curve" he had ever seen, and he advised a high protein diet with low fat. His future must have been in the hands of the Lord, as his faith had never waivered. He returned home and said, "I should be discouraged with that diagnosis — suspected cerebral arteriosclerosis — but I'm not. I have treated many patients with that, and that is not what I've got. However, that abnormal blood sugar curve interests me and I'm going to find out all I can about the opposite of diabetes."

It took a 4-month search to find out all he needed, but his recovery was very rapid when he got on the Seale Harris diet with no caffeine. Shots of . . . [trade name of calcium omitted] , combined with the other treatment of diet, helped to overcome his nervousness.

His recovery was like a miracle in our lives and was the answer to fervent prayers. Later, Dr. Gyland went to see the late Seale Harris to thank him for the discovery which saved his life. He also visited Dr. E. M. Abrahamson, and was intrigued by his dedication to an illness which many doctors ignore or treat with sugar.

All of my husband's symptoms disappeared and he had seven of the happiest and most productive years of his 35 years of practice. I helped him in the office, and it was a joy to us both to see alcoholics of thirty years standing get well, to see school children who were failing recover, postpartum cases get well. One man brought his wife in and said, "This is the last chance. If you can't help her, I'm getting a divorce. She is so irritable, I can't live with her any longer." When she had been under treatment only a few weeks, he told her, "I'm falling in love with you all over again." Her disposition changed radically and her asthma disappeared. Even when they returned to their home in Michigan, the severe winter did not bring on an attack, as she told us in Christmas cards over several years.

After an explanation of how the raw glands of the animals were prepared for feeding to allergic patients, the article continued as follows:

In nineteen children treated in the clinic and in nine adults institutionalized, we have not failed in a single instance to relieve the asthma. The children have almost universally been the type who have considerable bronchitis . . . The cortical hormone combined with epinephrin ointment has been quite effective in controlling eczema . . . It seems to be of value in migraine . . .

In discussing fifty cases of allergy patients treated with cortical extract and/or epinephrin, the physican stated:

The results of all but two were satisfactory. Neither of these patients was able to submit to a program of rest, which is so essential to the relief of their condition, but both patients experienced considerable increase in energy and a feeling of increased well-being, although neither was completely freed of the attacks . . . In speaking of relief we do not mean temporary relief, such as is obtained from a single injection of epinephrin, but a more permanent relief which leaves the patient free from symptoms.

The following pages are from this 1935 medical paper:

Table 1. – *Results of Treatment by the Use of Adrenal Hormones Administered Orally*

Type of Patient	Type of Therapy	Improvement			Total Number Patients
		Slight	Moderate	Marked	
In-patients	Epinephrin only	0	1	1	2
Out-patients	Epinephrin only	0	2	1	5
In-patients	Cortical extract only	0	0	1	1
Out-patients	Cortical extract only	0	0	2	2
Out-patients (children)	Epinephrine and cortical extract	0	7	12	19
Out-patients (adults)	Epinephrine and cortical extract	2	2	5	9
Out-patients (adults)	Epinephrine and cortical extract	0	6	4	10
In-patients	Miscellaneous therapy	0	0	2	2
		2	18	30	50

Three of adult in-patients treated less than two weeks. In each instance, relief of symptoms was obtained.

The following is typical of the type of children that we have been treating:

Case No. C-10434. — Male, aged eight years. Suffering from severe asthma. Treated with cortical extract and ep-inephrin orally, and a diet giving acid ash.

At the age of three years the patient suddenly developed asthma. He was given potassium iodine, ephedrin, also lactose, Maltine, and cod-liver oil, with no appreciable effect. In the spring of 1932 he was found sensitive to 57 of 300 antigens. He was given treatment without relief. In 1933 his asthma became worse, and in December was extremely distressing. His attacks were usually preceded by colds and were accompanied by severe coughing and wheezing. The attacks were milder during the summer and more severe during the winter. He gave a history of having little energy and always complained of being tired.

Examination revealed a red-haired, pale-skinned child of the angiospastic pseudo-anemic type. He had hypertrophied tonsils and enlargement of the cervical lymph glands. His chest showed many rhonchi and rales throughout, and was markedly emphysematous. The x-ray showed increased linear markings radiating from the hilum, suggestive of chronic bronchitis. Calcified nodes were present within the hilum on both sides.

A diagnosis of chronic asthma, with bronchitis, was made.

Although the patient had several colds, after treatment was begun they were less intense. After treatment began, February 10, 1934, he did not have a single paroxysm of asthma. During the first half of the school year, 1933-1934, he had missed school nearly half of the time, on account of colds and asthma. During the second half he lost only two weeks, and during the year of 1934-1935, he did not lose a single day of schooling. Previously he was unable to play with other children; but now he is interested in athletics and is a leader in sports, and it is with the greatest difficulty that he is kept from playing too hard. Severe physical exertion brings on coughing spells. During the eighteen months under treatment he has gained fourteen pounds, and his physical condition is excellent.

The use of ground adrenals prior to 1935 for relief of allergies reminds me of the use of ground liver in the 1920s, when liver was found to be a cure for the then-fatal pernicious anemia, also known as Addison's anemia.

As I studied this remarkable report made many years ago, I was thankful that I did not have to swallow a ground-up mixture of raw beef adrenal gland and peanut butter to be cured of my allergies. Apparently, in 1935 little was known about the high protein, low carbohydrate diet now being used with adrenal cortex extract in the treatment of allergy cases.

Dr. Sam E. Roberts, distinguished medical writer and former professor of Otolaryngology at the University of Kansas medical school, in his introduction to the first edition of *Goodbye Allergies,* said:

> "Judge Blaine has emphasized the constitutional approach to allergy — an approach which most physicians, especially the allergists, have failed to even recognize as a possible therapeutic tool in the management of allergy. The reason for this failure is that clinical nutrition is not taught in our medical schools. This book is a paradox in medical education, for it has the intelligent layman teaching the physician fundamental facts about nutrition . . . Every person who has any type of allergy, mild or debilitating, should read this book. Every practicing physician

should have the book in his private library. He should read
it with an open mind . . ."

In his latest medical book, *Exhaustion: Causes
and Treatment,** Dr. Roberts said he nominated me for
the "front row of the *Allergy Hall of Fame.*" He
said of *Goodbye Allergies:* "This book has done more
to inform the public than all the writings by the
entire medical profession on the subject of *allergy.*"

Dr. Roberts went on to say that he had treated
allergic patients for years with the treatment outlined
in my book, had talked with other physicians who
had successfully used the treatment with thousands
of patients, and all agreed that it was the safest and
most effective method for treatment of allergies.

Since the treatment discussed in the preceding
chapters can be used effectively for allergics of all
ages, the future of the allergic child is much brighter than it has been in the past. An allergic child is
usually an unhappy child. The parents and the child
have emotional problems they can't solve and which
make the allergies worse.

In the divorce courts, I have talked with scores of
small allergic children (usually asthmatics), who
actually had feelings of guilt over their parents'
marriage breakups.

It is not difficult to understand why a child has
such a guilt complex when a mother says, in the
presence of her children, "Then to add to all of my
problems, Jane started having asthmatic attacks."
It never once occurred to this self-pitying mother

* *Exhaustion: Causes and Treatment,* © Sam E. and Mary F. Roberts
Foundation, with permission of Radale Press.

that the parents' actions and conduct could produce enough emotional trauma to make any small, susceptible child asthmatic.

Many doctors tell parents of allergic children to treat their sons and daughters as if they were normal and healthy children. That, however, is frequently impossible, for if an allergic child is sent outdoors to play in the snow with the same amount of clothing worn by other children, the chances are he will get bronchitis or pneumonia. If he gets some kind of infection, even an ordinary cold, in the fall, he sometimes will have difficulty getting over it all winter.

When parents understand how important it is that allergic children suffer no unnecessary emotional upsets and that children can be cured of allergies by diet and medication, much of childhood's unhappiness will be prevented. Since the psychologists tell us the unhappy child will be the unhappy adult, it is imperative that our allergic children be cured of their allergies while they are still young. I know from experience the tragedy of being a sickly child. I never heard of the word "allergy" until I was grown. In my childhood there was little that could be done for allergies except to try to make the best of a bad situation. Thank God, children are now living in the age of medical miracles.

Nearly every day I get a letter or telephone call from some reader asking if I am still in good health. On my eightieth birthday my blood pressure was 124 over 70 and my weight is the same as it was when I entered military service in World War I.

Although retired from the bench, I accept court assignments from the Supreme Court. This editorial appeared late in 1975 in the Kingfisher, Oklahoma, *Times*: "Judge Tom R. Blaine has just completed six weeks of district court assignment in this county. The judge, who writes books on nutrition, is the best advertisement for his books. He looks, acts and thinks like a man 30 years younger than he is."

In December, 1975, I visited with a physician friend I had not seen in 35 years. He remarked: "When I treated you in the late thirties I didn't think you would live to be 60. You don't look that old now."

Some allergists tell patients that the plan of treatment discussed in this book was found to be worthless and discarded years ago. More than 100 doctors have told me this statement is false and made to deceive.

If your physician desires information on adrenal cortex extract, I suggest he write Adrenal Metabolic Research Society of Hypoglycemia Foundation, P.O. Box 98, Fleetwood, Mt. Vernon, N.Y. 10552.

Please don't ask me to help you find a doctor. If I knew the name and address of a physician in your city who had prescribed the medication I recommend, I would not give you that information. You might show my letter to another physician who would claim to a medical association the doctor was using a layman to get patients. Anything a physician tells me will always remain confidential.

If you are unable to find a local physician who is interested in helping you get over your allergies, you might inquire of either:

1. International Academy of Preventative Medicine, 871 Frostwood Drive, Houston, Texas 77024.

2. International College of Applied Nutrition, Box 386, La Habra, California 90631.

3. International Academy of Metabiology, 2236 Suree Ellen Lane, Altadena, California 91001.

To get an answer you will have to be specific in your request and enclose a self-addressed, stamped envelope.

If a doctor tells you that adrenal cortical extract is a form of cortisone, ask him to read the label of a bottle of the extract where it says it is manufactured from the adrenals of young domestic animals.

Over 80 per cent of those who wrote me about their marvelous recoveries from allergies said the only medical help they had was from local (usually family) physicians.

Always remember these things:

1. Hypoglycemia, or low blood sugar, is as much a nutritional disease as is diabetes.

2. Glucose tolerance tests are routinely given in hospitals and in most physicians' offices.

3. Unless the anti hypoglycemia diet lessens the severity of your allergies, you should not incur the expense of adrenal cortex extract treatments.

Speaking in the language of my profession, the law, this new method of treating and curing allergic sufferers needs no advocates to plead its cause before the tribunals of modern medicine. It is entitled to impartial, unbiased, and fair hearings before the supreme court of medicine — the physicians of the nation. Whenever and wherever it has been fairly, honestly, and competently tried, the results have been so much better than were anticipated that it has already been proven to be a miracle of modern medicine.